Having Babies Over 40

A Humorous Glimpse at Pregnancy and Parenthood Later in Life

By Jacqueline Ramirez

Chapter Guide

		Page
Part 1 Getting Pregnant		
1	Pregnancy Books and Advice.	1
2	#Trending#Lateinlife(LIL)Mommies Or For You D&D Fans #Rolling A 100 Sided Die.	16
3	Getting Knocked Up. Clean Up Your Act And Get Laid.	20
4	Confused Ladies And Calling Your Doctor. C'me On Man!	29
5	Who's House? Run's House. Paging Dr. 'Cover Yo Ass.'	33
Part 2 Pregnant? Now What?		
6	McSteamy, Nurse Ratchet And Dealing With Insurance.	43
7	Take Off All Of Your Clothes And Put On This Paper Towel.	48
8	Testing and Screenings. Are We Having Fun Yet?	60
9	Weight Gain. Reaching Goodyear Blimp Status.	67
10	Our Loss. Baby Grace.	73
11	Everybody Has Something.	83
12	I Know All There Is To Know About The Gender Game.	85
13	"We" Are Pregnant, Aka Your Husband Is An Idiot.	87
14	Finding the Perfect Father.	90
15	Naming Your Child.	92
16	Eating Godzilla Style.	93
17	Yoga. Not Just For Hipsters And Old Ladies.	101
18	Basic Whining And Complaints.	104
19	The Fear is Real and the Anxiety Overwhelming.	108
Part 3 Having a Baby. OMG is this For Real?		
20	Packing For The Hospital.	111
21	It Just Got Real Round 1. Full Moon On Friday The 13[th.]	116
22	It Just Got Real Round 2. Natural Childbirth And The Ring Of Fire.	120
23	L&D Game FAQs Player Game Walk Thru.	128
24	My Best Delivery Room Advice.	148
25	General Comments For The Aftermath.	150
26	Things I Was Surprised By.	157
Part 4 After Baby. And Now the Fun Begins.		
27	Sunday Bloody Funbag Funday.	162
28	Sex And The Scene Of The Crime.	169
29	Stretch Marks, Leaky Bladders and Gas, Oh My.	175
30	Good Luck with that Baby Weight, Bitch.	182
31	Your Baby's New Home.	189

Chapter Guide Continued

		Page
32	Stay At Home Mom Guidelines.	193
33	#TripleP-PukePoopPeeImmunity #Break Out Your HazMatSuit.	199
34	The Stickiest Of the Icky. 2x the kids = clean up x 100.	209
35	But It's Supposed to be About ME!!!	213
36	Ever Changing Moods.	215
37	When I Get Some Sleep.	217
38	Waylaid By Jackassary.	219
39	How To Still Be YOU And Be A Parent.	223
40	Unsolicited Advice. The Scourge of New Mom Existence.	226
41	And Now MY 2 Cents On Some Hot Button Topics Aka Some Unsolicited Advice.	232
42	Fidgety Parents. It's Torture.	236
43	Mind Set of Being a LIL (Late in Life) Mon and Dealing with Ancient Grandparents.	239
44	Wrap It Up!	241

Part 5 Buying Guide

45	What Do You Really Need To Bring Baby Home? And my 2 cents on baby items.	246

Part 1 Getting Pregnant

1. Pregnancy Books And Advice.

My husband's catch phrase is go write a blog about it. Along the same lines a quote from Chelsea Handler in response to someone who was writing a book but didn't have a publisher yet, and she said 'honey then it's a blog not a book.' I thought about writing a blog then I referenced my less than exciting but all together time consuming experience with pregnancy books. Between my mom and husband and friends I was gifted and bought about 30 different books and DVD's. Ranging from late in life pregnancies, to general information to birth coaching and tips on breastfeeding. The best one I read was co-authored by Dr. Oz.

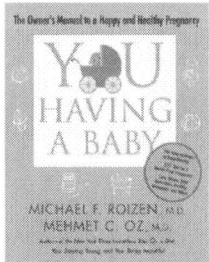

Schribner , SIMON & SCHUSTER

Straight forward, pretty good illustrations, and fairly informative, however but not as comprehensive as I needed. The rest really meander. I seriously wanted to be able to flip to the index and read about a specific issue, ailment, developmental stage or just to ease my mind at 2am when the panic and anxiety took over. I wanted fast, hard medical answers. Well my book isn't from a medical standpoint, just my story. I was over 40 when I started trying and a few months shy of 46 when I had my last baby. I'm informed. I read a lot. Between the dozens of books, I also subscribed to several web site communities, had ½ a dozen apps on my phone to reference at any given time and read hundreds of articles. It's cliché but everyone and every pregnancy is different so no one source fits all of your needs. Even with the gluttony of data I found some of my best and worst resources to be the people around me. My prenatal yoga instructor is also a doula and a Bradley method expert. She was to the point and had simple home cures for most pregnancy ailments including my painfully swollen feet and ankles during month 8. One of my best friends is super smart and determined and knowledgeable and tenacious. Another friend is opinionated with a ton of life experience. Add to that the myriad of relatives and strangers who want to throw their 2 cents in the mix and I wasn't at a loss for people telling me what I should and shouldn't do, how I should and shouldn't act, what I should and shouldn't be feeling or just to goose me with some horror story about how hard things are going to be or to sweep in with some smarmy comment about I was going to look back at my current discomfort and laugh because there is a world of shit descending on me hadn't even started yet. Now I am a confident person. Not one easily swayed by others or peer pressure and I found myself at times riddled with doubt from the overwhelming onslaught of unsolicited advice and dramatic scare tactics type pregnancy warnings. Coupled with three high risk pregnancies I was lucky to keep my sanity.

BTW congratulations if you are expecting or expecting to be expecting soon. Mazel Tov. Always always always congratulate a pregnant woman, but make sure she is pregnant first and not just having a bloated day or a food baby. And mean it with the most absolute sincerity. As you will find being pregnant is like being at war, and while it seems sweet that almost everyone wants to sop and talk to you or even touch your belly, not everyone has something nice to say. In fact most have some nasty story to pass on that is usually scary, miserable or just depressing about their birth experience or that of a close friend, or better yet a judgment about how fat or how not fat you are. So if you see someone you know is having a baby, and confirm this by having them tell you that yes they are expecting, congratulate them on their impending joy and tell them they are glowing and look fabulous and you are so happy for them. Most importantly stop there. No additional story or detail about your pregnancy is needed. Every child is a blessing. Well most. Ok some. Well mainly just mine. Another lesson to learn is that if you didn't like babies or kids before, you still won't, you will just like your own.

Being pregnant is like becoming famous. All of sudden there is a peak in social interest. There is a lot of doctoring and advice being thrown around by those who've seen it. Everyone has your solution and answers to your problems. Truthfully advice is only as good as your frame of mind in wanting to accept it or having a specific problem it addresses. I have a friend who's father in law used to boast about his girlfriend's grandchild. The parents are very much stereotypical Millennials and have specific diets and child raising philosophies. Everyone in their household was on a very strict macrobiotic diet, and still nursing their first baby until she was 48 months old (that's 4 to regular folks.) He used to joke that he and his girlfriend were thinking of calling social services on them because everyone looked pale, emaciated, and way too thin. They also utilized various behavior techniques that included never saying "no" as well as refraining from yelling or raising their voices. Now when pressed this grandpa had to admit that my friends weren't using any specific child raising method or school of thought. "Just like normal," he would tell his girlfriend's super educated friends and adult children. The family ended up having another baby and all hell broke loose with their latest arrival. The first born got very jealous, and their world and rules and techniques were shook to the ground. All of the methods backfire a little at some point. I'm taking a very 'organic' approach which is code for I'm too frickin' tired to set up very strict regimens for my kid and too resource poor at this time to enroll my 3 year old in school or have him in daycare so he's with me and I'm just watching him evolve and grow and learn while I take care of my 10 month old. So I guess just raising them "normal." You will find that routines and patterns develop as does a tolerance for behaviors that you will and won't live with. As you get more kids, inevitably the more structure comes about due to you having to be more organized to manage your growing hoard. As a wise woman once said, there are ladies who squat in rice paddies and pop out babies and go back to work. Women used to have babies in caves. Many women think or find that basic parenting is an innate ability. I took to it pretty naturally and found my instincts kicked in on a lot of day to day tasks and issues. Some women have it, some don't, and sometimes your husband is the better parent.

With becoming a parent you also become and uber consumer of baby and subsequently kid 'stuff.' All of the extras and ancillary 'necessities' are just marketing and sales pitches at some point. I must say I've been very skeptical over the years about the 'expiration' date on car seats, though I don't question the value and necessity of their use one bit, it's the whole notion that it expires like milk that gets me. No you don't want a car seat that has been in an accident and taken a severe impact, but expire? Like after a certain date it doesn't work anymore? I'm still not sure about that. Feels very much like it is all about money and marketing. You will start watching kids TV and I just read a factoid today that Ronald Reagan signed off on a law allowing advertising and product placement in programming directed at children that in part funded and fostered what we see today. Very good shows, excellent shows that hook our kids in and teach them some solid basic skills but all sell sell sell to your kids so hardcore that every commercial break in our house is followed by a Oh My GOD I need that. To which I cleverly reply 'put it on your Christmas list" or "tell nana." Having a baby is a Hallmark holiday on crack and they got you coming and going. Not only do you need copious amounts of supplies while you are pregnant, you need even more after the baby comes and if you don't buy the best of the best of the best you are a bad and negligent parent. Well that's the way some of the advertising mumbo jumbo and the emotions it summons makes you feel. There are only a few things that you need the best on, very few, surprisingly few.

During your pregnancy you are expected at minimum to purchase the following:
Prenatal vitamins. You need them so just do it and start before you conceive to build up your folic acid levels. Everyone on the planet agrees that increasing your folic acid levels helps reduce birth defects so just do it. If you are older this is a no brainer and bypassing the vitamins isn't worth one more extra risk added on top of the insurmountable road you have in front of you. Find a brand you can live with and stomach and do it. Everyday. Just do it. It's not that big of a deal. I see women complain about it all of the time, just suck it up and do it. Yes it sucks feeling like crap and queasy and then taking a vitamin that may also make you burp up

yuckiness and feel like crap and queasy. You are cooking a human being, learn to sacrifice your comfort even a little already.

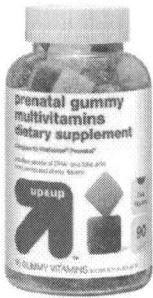

Target.com Up & Up Brand

I recommend Target generic brand prenatal vitamins either caplet form or the gummy. If you read the labels they have all of the same ingredients as the $30 a bottle vitamins from the more holistic food store. Also you can get free samples from your OB, they have a ton. You can send away on manufacture web sites and ask for samples, I think even Babies R Us gives you free samples with your baby registry goodie bag. Pretend you are an adult and take your vitamins already.

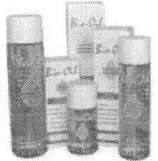

Bio-Oil

Bio-oil or Palmers for stretch marks. Oils and lotions to rub on your growing belly to reduce stretch marks is a pregnant woman's ritual. After you shower is a good time. My two cents however is that it doesn't work and you either get stretch marks because it's your genetics or the nature of your skin or you won't. I've gained a ton of weight and lost a ton of weight over the past few years and I don't have a single stretch mark. Ha ha suckers, but seriously it's just my skin. I'm 47 and I look 37 and I don't take any extraordinary measures to stay looking young, I'm blessed with good skin. I was gifted a few bottles of bio-oil as well as a bottle of stretch mark oil from the health food store. I used it all at some point, if not on my skin on my kid's skin. It's decent but I can't say that anything prevents stretch marks. You have my sympathy if you do get bad stretch marks. You can reduce the appearance quite a bit by using self tanner on the area, it makes them disappear camouflage style.

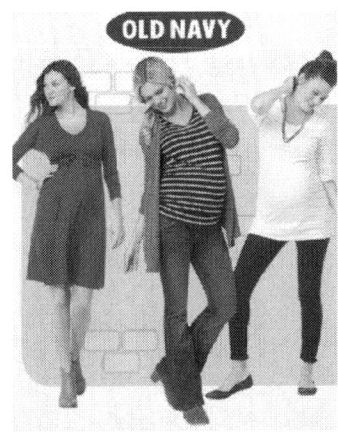

Old Navy.com, Gap Inc.

Maternity clothes. Now there is some very very cute stuff out there and during my first pregnancy I went nuts and bought dresses and tops and jeans and all kinds of awesome cute clothes. It's hard to resist. It's so exciting. I recommend Old Navy. Their clothes aren't built to last but who cares you will want to throw them away afterwards anyway. No one wants to have to have their maternity jeans linger around after delivery. Kohl's isn't bad either. Target is ok, the clothes themselves aren't that great but their return policies and the fact that they have everything else you will ever need for your kids for the first 10 years or so is quite a draw. But hey it's not about style it's about comfort right? I have a friend who's kids are now teenagers. She was pregnant in the Midwest and said she went to the local goodwill and bought black stretch pants and big sweatshirts. One of my dear friends borrowed her husbands tee's and sweats towards the end. I stayed pretty true to what worked for me and I wore it to death. Shortly after my last baby I did a complete and cathartic purge on my closet. The ultimate irony was that my yoga pants that I pushed to the max over and over again actually gave out in the inner thigh seam during a prenatal yoga class. One big rip. C'est la vie. Now there are pieces you are going to wear ALL of the time and some you will put on a time or two and those are the ones that usually cost the most. Stretchy black t-shirt, $15. Lovely maternity blouse to wear once to a brunch, $60. After the giddiness of my first pregnancy wore off I really wore the following: A very springy and generous pair of yoga pants, well several. A plain black semi fitted t-shirt that was so super comfortable and looked decent because it was fitted and grew with me as I got bigger. You need to flatter the girls who will be up front and fabulous. Put a spot light on them. Now your bump and dealing with pants are a whole different story. All eyes will be on your boobs and belly so unless you are a supermodel the key for the bottom area is camouflage with either a dark maternity jean or black yoga pants. A long black jersey skirt is a plus too for those days that adulting and pants are just too much.

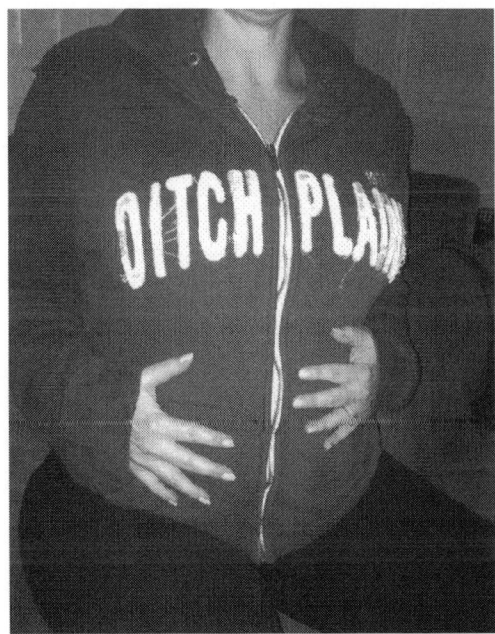

Stolen oversized super warm sweateshirt

I also needed a few large zip hoodies. When I got cold it was a bad scene. I would shake uncontrollably and feel almost paralyzed. A very large zip hoodie is your friend when you are knocked up. Steal that from your husbands closet or in my case I stole one from my husband that he had stolen from his friend. These guys were former football players and the friend lives in a cold climate so it was big and warm. Yummy. We let him know it had been stolen when my husband sent him a picture of a very pregnant me snuggled up in it. I bought a few dresses and slacks and nice tops and rarely broke them out across 3 pregnancies. Stick with what works and what you feel good in.

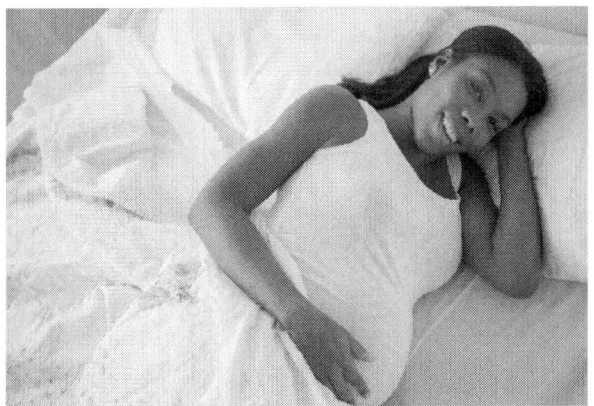

Photo from SheKnows.com

Nice Bedding. Ok we don't need to break the bank here so not too nice but you will want to seed your nest and the sanctuary of your bed with lots of comfy pillows and blankets. If you don't buy new ones bust out all of your highest quality bedding and set it up. At minimum you will need ½ a dozen pillows, and 2 blankets for when you feel cold and a nice crisp cool top sheet for when you are hot. If it's your first, and for some ladies your only pregnancy, that bed is going to be your best friend. Offering more comfort than you husband or a candy bar. You will want to sleep, sleep, nap, sleep and sleep some more. Get it all in. Sleep the deepest most peaceful sleep of you life. If you have other kids around already, I suggest locking the door but seriously before you have more kids the sleep of your first pregnancy is like no other. So spruce up your bed a little. Consider getting some bed accessories like a sleep mask or one of those scented eye pillows. Maybe even some aromatherapy spray. Think spa and sanctuary and even after the baby comes you may be surprised how much time you end up spending in that bed so make it look and smell nice.

Smart Phone. If you don't have one already I guess I would ask what is wrong with you, but I'll cut everyone some slack. Gone are the days of the regular camera, and even the digital camera has become extinct. You can blast to the past when hospitals or doctors used to give expectant fathers a pager so their partner could page them if they were going into labor. How Doogie Howser. You will need a phone to do the following pregnant activities: shop on line for all of your baby stuff, Google all of your symptoms and check out all of the baby name sites, and to take pictures of your crazy meals and pregnant selfies to post of your blog. The same blog you will abandon at some point because life will catch up with you and you will find its easier just to text pictures of your new little one to your family and friends and post them on FaceBook and Instagram instead of maintaining an actual blog. So you will need a smart phone to take a jillion pictures of your new baby, edit them and send them off. You might as well go ahead and add about a hundred apps. Shopping sites like Target and Babies R Us (which BTW is a crap site and is slower and more clumsy than you will have the patience to deal with) as well as some miscellaneous blogs and registry sites. Then add your ovulation and due date apps. Those are fun figuring out what your due date is if you get pregnant at your next opportunity. You'll need access to the millions of potential baby names so you can start clocking in the hours upon hours searching for that perfect name and to secretly laugh at and judge all of the super popular names as well as the insane names some celebrities come up with. You can add the "What to Expect When You're Expecting" app so you can get weekly growth information about you and the baby, as well as access to their boards to read and post about all of your pregnancy related thoughts. Nothing says I'm hormonal and crazy than obsessively trolling pregnancy posts to viciously respond to at 3am. You are also are going to need something to watch in bed at 2am, both before and after the baby comes so download what works for you, if it's Netflix, Hulu, HBO Now or U-verse. I must add that while pregnant I got hooked on Keeping Up With The Kardashians as well as repeats of the Jersey Shore on MTV. So good. So yummy.

The obligatory pregnancy books and videos. As fore mentioned I have quite a few. I did read them all. And here I am penning my very own because they and this are woefully incomplete. I think you need to really know the medical basics. How to conceive. Yes there are folks out there who have no real clue how it works outside of sperm and egg and don't understand the timing of ovulation and fertility windows etc. I'm completely shocked every time I talk to a woman over 40 who is toying around with the notion of having a baby that they have no idea what an ovulation monitor is and how to track the fertility windows. Essential for most women but especially after 40 when you do NOT have time to screw around, well you do and you don't right, you don't have time to waste, how's that. You need to know matter of fact what happens after conception and the basic anatomical development of your baby as well as the physical changes to you. How you exist as one system for 9 months. I think you need some insight into the potential negative aspects like the bad physical symptoms, as well as the potentially dangerous developmental problems for your baby. What are borderline symptoms and what are warning signs that something is wrong. I had bleeding with one of my pregnancies, and the cause was a uterine tear. No one wants to get scared but you need to be informed enough to be able to ask the right questions. The more you know the more you have to worry about but you can always bring a list of questions into your doctor and call your doctors nurse at anytime. They really expect that you are going to be nervous and have a million questions to call anytime and ask, that is what they are there for. It's hard to be pregnant and start to understand how much you don't know. It's vast what you don't know. It's overwhelming what you don't know. But suck it up ladies, it only gets harder after this. Nothing worth having is easy as they say. Finally I think you need to see someone who is celebrating this amazing miracle and for some the best period of their lives. It's beyond anything else that I've ever experienced and I find myself wistfully nostalgic about my pregnancies and deliveries. It's beyond words even going through this most precious life event, and one who if you are around or close to my age you waited a really long time to experience and it's even more magical and wonderful than anyone could ever describe to you.

What I found most valuable out of all of the advice and books and blogs was the following;

> Knowing what to expect. Hence "What To Expect When You're Expecting." Everyone is different. I kind of wish someone would write a book called things are going to get out of control, here are some crazy ass things that will happen. I talk to new moms all of the time who seem taken aback or surprised by some of the changes to their bodies and things their kids do.

> How many doctor appointments and what they were going to entail. I've had more vials of blood drawn, tests administered and hands inside my lady parts than I can bear to remember.

> How to overcome problems like feeling like crap for 9 months. I found myself during my last pregnancy taking more medication than I had in the prior 10 years. I had Krakatau magnitude acid reflux and heartburn that depleted my daily life so dramatically and without prescription acid reducers I couldn't function.

> What to buy ahead of time and what to pack for the hospital. When your brain function starts to shrivel up and die you need a check list for that bag. You won't use 70% of what you pack but that stuff you need you REALLY need so over-packing isn't the problem it's remembering the important stuff.

> You need advice on actually laboring and having a baby. Everyone will tell you something different.

> What baby items to buy, what to really invest in, and what to take a pass on. As 'Mericans we are completely over commercialized. Don't think for a second there aren't people sitting in a room inventing items that we 'must' buy and creating marketing materials for those 'must' buy items so they can get

rich. Women in 3rd world countries make it work without the latest swaddling blankets and rock-a-bye electronic cradles.

> Dealing with that first year. My eyes are burning just remembering the sleep deprivation and insanity.

> How involved your husband should be. It's all about you and your comfort level but seriously you aren't going to watch the video tape of the birth at a later time so take a pass on that nonsense. You'd probably like your husband to be enticed into having sex with you again after that 6 week mark, even with no sleep trust me you are going to want that sex more than any sex you've ever had. So less is more as they say. The less he sees that could shun him away from touching you down there ever again the better.

> Breastfeeding. Uggggh it really hurts at first. I read a book that talked about positions and exclusively breastfeeding or else it would get all screwed up. I didn't exclusively nurse with my son, but I did with my daughter. Does it make a difference? Yes it truly does but as with all of this it boils down to one simple frustrating phrase.

You have to experience it to understand it. It is the awful truth. I've had a medicated and drug free birth experience. I could have read a million books and talked to a million women and having a 'natural' birth is the most intense experience I've ever had in my life and nothing prepared me for it. Being informed gave me the ability to squash my terror and panic at a given moment but truthfully didn't make it any easier or keep my head on any straighter. The only thing that helped was having gone through the process, even once, to have some basis of comparison and to know that you aren't going to die or accidentally give birth in a toilet or the car on the way to the hospital.

At our advanced age, you want your pregnancy to be in a stress free bubble. Good luck. It's nearly impossible given our stage of life and the enormous risks. So it would seem only the 20 year old accidentally pregnant after only dating for a few months with their parents to fall back on and some kind of magic money cloud get to live in that bubble. For the rest of us it's rough. In an anxiety reducing precaution, please beware of social media trolls on pregnancy forums. I did so much reading while I was pregnant the first two times. From books to blogs, to daily postings. My data consumption was as large as my appetite. My husband always says trust none of what you hear and half of what you see. Could not hold more true for on line pregnancy forums. The woefully misinformed have launched a social media platform that provides very little real information, very little support and like most media is somewhat entertaining. There are daily fights and I mean knock down drag out name calling fights. I found myself caught up in the fray between my surging hormones and raging anxiety and doubt I spent precious time and energy weighing in on opinions and topics that were trivial and my contribution wasn't going to gain anyone anything other than to give someone more pissed off than I was fuel to fire back at me with. I guess the tenants of Christianity are checked at the door when you sign up on one of these forums. Being kind and having compassion are erased by making sure your opinion is voiced. One of the life lessons I've learned in my 45+ years, and it was hard learned, was its sometimes better to be polite than right. I know in my heart that I'm right on a lot of counts and I'm self aware enough to understand when I need assistance or don't have the answers. Well don't argue with an angry pregnant 20 year old who has an opinion on everything from gestational diabetes to baby shower gifts. I found myself trying to help by offering up stories and opinions based on my experiences and my knowledge base. You don't get pregnant after 40 by accident and you don't go in not knowing some of the odds and statistics. I became a punching bag like every other contributor on the pregnancy sites and had to finally remove myself in my 8th month because it was too overwhelming and would spike my blood pressure to read some of the responses. It was also highly addicting and I found myself logging on all of the time and constantly reading my own posts and the responses to them, waiting for some thank you's or some indication that I helped someone which came far too infrequently. Having said that websites and communities are helpful, like the Mayo clinic, WebMD, etc. but take them with a grain of salt please. Very few if any experts are posting. Just moms with their own two cents. Some of which are very rude and judgmental.

I was on an online community and got involved in a string on breastfeeding. I had a ton of problems getting going with my son and supplemented him with bottles from the get go. I enjoyed that my husband could give me a break and get some bonding in by bottle feeding him and it was the best solution for us as a family at the time. Exclusively nursing takes your husband out of the equation really unless you want to pump and put it in a bottle which trust me you are probably going to be too tired and sore to do. I posted my two cents and got BLASTED unmercifully about being a hack and giving out poor advice and being a bad parent. F you too bitchy website posters. Be warned. On line communities serve a purpose but so many haters and trollers make them prohibitive especially while pregnant sensitive and vulnerable.
So you think a book is safer but most pregnancy books are either blandly informative or lame and repetitive. Ironically what I disliked in other pregnancy books I believe I'm replicating here. I wanted facts, I wanted information, I wanted to be able to look up a word in the index and it would take me to a page with the answer. This is not that. This are my stories about my 3 pregnancies over the age of 40 that allowed me to have a wide circle of experience. Also the trials and challenges of the first few years raising these beings that just shot out of my body. I want to include situations and advice that I didn't come across in the other books I've read. There doesn't seem to be much middle ground. As a stay at home mom I talk to a lot of ladies in my neighborhood about their experiences. We all have gone through the same thing but it can be so much different and individual just as every pregnancy that you have is unique and has different pluses and minuses. Different things that you love and hate, and if you can survive it all and have a healthy baby and not be a twisted mess of neurosis and not "accidentally" kill your husband when he's driving you nuts then we are truly all in the same boat and we need to stick together. Solidarity ladies so let's get to it. To clear the slate too, this book isn't just for older moms or traditional family configurations, if you have a cooch, a fetus and a funny bone then I'm talking to you. As similar as all of our general experiences

are, the details can be very different. It's going to get graphic as giving birth and raising babies is a messy explosion of body fluids. I also want to make you laugh. There is no greater magic than being able to make your kids laugh. I kind of learned that from the dog whisperer, that you need to realign dogs, I mean kids, when they aren't acting right and he does it by a snap or a tap on the nape of the neck or a nudge on their side. I will touch my child either on the arm or the back and I will try to tell a joke or do something stupid or funny to get them to laugh. When they are mad, or sad, or tired, or angry if you can figure out how to change the mood and make you kids laugh, it's gold. I hope it does the same for you, to reduce any anxiety or stress you are having as your miracle and blessing is getting ready to meet the world.

2. #Trending #Lateinlife(LIL)Mommies Or For You D&D Fans #Rolling A 100 Sided Die.

The number of women having babies over 40 has increased significantly, exponentially over the last 30 years, a trend that will continue into the next decades. The good news is that teen pregnancy is trending significantly down, and women are waiting longer and longer to have children. Why?

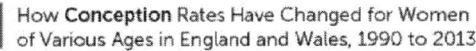

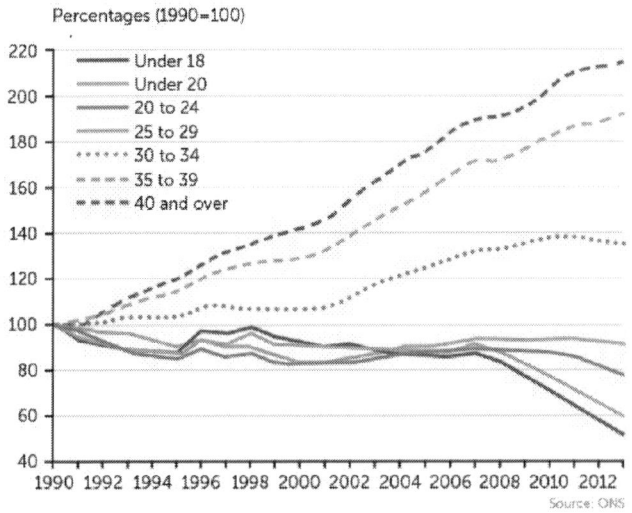

The split in the 70's between motherhood and career has been abolished. The growing pains of the 80's and 90's with the concept of having to be Supermom has been equalized by husbands and father's stepping up to the plate. Not to be underestimated is the adjustment of the mindset in our culture that babies are cool. Men not only are excited about being parents but many are taking over the traditional mommy duties and being stay at home dads and I know a few they are super cool and love their roles and I love that. There is nothing like seeing a father with his little girl. It melts your heart. We also have a mindset that employers should accommodate women having children and that public nursing is a right. Society has now put a premium on having babies which is an offshoot of the 00's trend of carrying a small dog everywhere you went. Being pregnant is fab and with women's rights and job protected it's a path that offers personal reward. I also have to believe that the notion 20-30 years ago that if you were pregnant you could potentially lose your job has given way to the philosophy that maybe we shouldn't discount ½ our population because they breed. That making more people is a natural state. Having sex is good and makes people happy. Having kids is good and makes people feel fulfilled. Sink or swim, and currently our culture has chosen to swim, and embrace parenthood and the necessity of parents to do their best. Raising happy smart capable children has been made a priority as the adverse effect of not doing so has been felt in drug abuse and crime rates. It's a genesis of our society that happy people procreating is becoming a very very Martha Stewart 'good thing.' How do we reduce the issues that plague us and bring us down? We educate and raise our children properly and are given the adequate resources to do so. We start from a place of love and acceptance and put our focus into the happiness, stability and daily joy of our family unit. Happy people make happy kids.

Soap box preaching aside, what I've done over the last few years by having 2 kids over 40 is going to become an ever popular stance. I'm mature, patient, informed, financially more secure and I have a desire to have and raise children. Now a days there really isn't as much stigma on being pregnant as there is on NOT being pregnant. It's expected when you make the decision to either seriously couple up or yikes get married. I think people feel more informed about partnering up and getting married now a days. It's almost as if all of the divorces and choosing to live together instead of getting married has made the commitment to actually take the plunge more serious. With the accepted choice of not having children gaining popularity as well, the push on those who do want children and a family is being moved to the forefront. Getting married implies a very serious and intense commitment and children are almost always expected, so kind of old school but with new eyes. If you want kids have them in abundance. If you love kids and have a good marriage or partnership and your partner loves kids, sign you up to have a few. If you don't, then don't. It's equally as cool now a days not to procreate.

The celebrity set has made all pregnancies but especially those later in life look like a piece of cake. Get pregnant, gain a little weight or a lot depending on you, work you ass off to get the weight off and get paid twice; once for having a baby photo shoot with your new bundle of joy and a few months later landing the cover of a magazine in a bikini showing off your post baby figure. Then you get become a baby expert, write a blog, put your name on some baby food and baby clothes and rake it in. Babies are the new dogs. Everyone has one, and if you don't have one you want one and they are big business. I never realized how having a baby did make me part of a special and very exclusive club and that club really revolves around the age of your baby. Moms of newborns are in a different tier than those with toddlers, than those with school age kids, etc. etc. At these club meetings you trade stories about pregnancy and kids. You also brag a bit and panic can ensue as you hear about how this child can do this already etc. I have women in my peer group who had kids reading and writing at 3. I've come to understand this is a dynamic that will continue until, forever. There will always be someone who's child is bigger, faster, stronger, smarter. But it doesn't matter. What matters is you and your child, the love and the relationship. All kids even out at some point and I'm so glad we live in a time where being 'normal' isn't the desired state of affairs anymore. Being different and being an individual is where it's at. One of the cool things about being a LIL (late in life) mom is that you are too tired and too far down the road to give a crap most days. I don't brag on my children, much. It isn't my thing. My family is originally from the east coast so that dry sense of humor has you telling self deprecating stories more than trading my kids are better than yours statistics. Truthfully, I'm so old that my dad and my kids now need the same amount of care. They need diapers, constant feeding, they whine and drool.

Lastly let's not forget the technology that gives people who are reproductively challenged greater options. That's what moves those numbers around the most for women over 40 having babies. The medical know how to generate and sustain a pregnancy in less than optimal conditions. Coupled with people like me, who successfully became pregnant and had perfect kids after 40, even

45, helps move the statistics in a positive direction for us later in life parents. And most are not just to have one baby, but multiples with lots and lots of sets of twins as a result of fertilizing several embryos and implanting more than one at a time. In about 10 years twins will be a norm in High School. A calling card for my parents had a problem having babies so they used external measures. Our teachers are going to have to take classes on how to manage multiples in their classrooms. A very new concept. Not just a good friend but a sibling to get in trouble with and potentially an identical sibling. Like teachers don't have enough problems to navigate and on pauper wages to boot. The multiple revolution is going to hit our society hard as these kids go through the public school systems and move into adulthood and we will have to adjust. Educators will have to take mandated classes about how to cope and be 'sensitive' to the twin dynamic.

At the end of the day babies are good. Babies are a blessing. I see the difference in my peer group between the babies that were hard fought for and the ones that were an ooops. The hard fought for babies have their name in wooden letters adorning the wall of their perfectly painted and decorated nursery. The ooops end up in a used pack n play with hand me down gender indifferent clothing. I get that's a bold generalization. I fought for all of my kids even though I took a very practical approach to my baby product consumption. FYI babies can't really see so all of the up front nursery decoration and exquisite clothing choices are for you, not them.

3. Getting Knocked Up. Clean Up Your Act And Get Laid.

You will find everyone has a lot of different advice about how to get pregnant. You think you know but you don't. I had the good fortune of having a wonderful friend who was very well versed in all of the ins and outs, so to speak, of timing around ovulation and frequency of intercourse. She was also getting pregnant and having babies at the same time I wanted to. Ironically years prior when both of our husband horizons were bleak we talked about going to the sperm bank and buying the same sperm and having siblings. She ended up married and pregnant a few months before me and became my go to resource on impregnation. Her advice was to have sex the day before and the day after you ovulate. She cited some references that do tell you not to hit it too frequently because you will diminish the concentration of swimmers. I don't know about all of that, all I know is what worked for me. I was told by my regular doctor (GP), who had her first children at 40, a set of twins she had after years of treatments for infertility, the following: ***That if this was something I wanted to really do I needed to start preparing my body now.*** I needed to get in shape. I needed to cut out any partying. I need to start eating really well, add lots of antioxidants to my diet like blueberries and to start taking prenatal vitamins immediately to build up my folic acid levels. Finally she advised me to by a Clearblue easy ovulation monitor. They cost about $200 and the strips cost $50 a box.

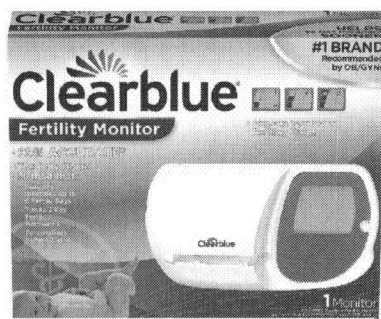

Clearblue ® Fertility Monitor

For the most part I followed her guidelines and have some insights of my own. **I suggest to immediately start using an ovulation**

monitor. Read and follow the directions and use it perfectly to the letter for at least two months to set your base line up right. To supplement this information download a few apps to help you with tracking and fertility windows. Don't waste time. You don't have it to waste. It can take months to gauge your fertility and years to get pregnant if you have problems. For most women who are facing challenges getting pregnant when they want to the 1st stage is Clomid (a drug that stimulates multiple eggs to drop during ovulation) and hormone injections, then IVF if that doesn't take and IVF is a long, difficult, costly and excruciating process that doesn't guarantee any results. You need to find out ASAP if you are viable, if you husband is making good swimmers and if your body is able to grow a baby. Well gathered information is the key. It's not romantic, in fact it's pretty sterile but getting as much knowledge as possible helps. You will have to be an adult and filter out things that aren't working for you or you feel you can't do. For example I never did a basal temperature baseline or tried to measure my temperature as an ovulation marker. The simplistic view is you pee on a stick to help track your hormones. When your body is ready the Clearblue Easy monitor has a little egg that shows up on the display which means 'now is the time to have sex.' Lots of sex. In a few weeks pee on a stick again. Done and done. It's not complicated but do yourself a favor and be as precise as possible to avoid error. To give you a range I ovulated about 11to 12 days after the first day of my period. Utilize whatever organization system, calendar app that works best for you, but you have to track the first day of your period and your ovulation dates in order to get a good window of fertility. I would have sex for the few days before and after ovulation. After sex I would linger in bed for about 5-10 minutes with my feet up in the air to try and keep all of the spermies moving in the right direction and inside me as long as possible. I don't think that helps but it made me feel like it was helping. Mind over matter is a serious factor in fertility. If you talk to couples who have had fertility issues they will tell you it isn't all cut and dry. Fertility changes, it isn't black and white, off or on. It's also a heartbreak every month when their period comes, especially after intense treatments like IVF. My heart goes out to any and everyone faced with these problems. They are not simple, they are expensive and stressful and really put you through the wringer. So many variables are at play and one of the main themes I've heard from my friends is that with a shift in mindset and a release from stress your body tends to respond more favorably. I know several couples who have benefited from acupuncture and massage therapy. I have a dear friend who after fertility treatments had a complete body reset, like the pregnancy taught her body what to do and it was able to function properly afterwards. So the fact that it made me feel much more confident when I laid on my back and put my feet towards the ceiling and I felt that I was increasing my chances to get an egg fertilized that perhaps that might have contributed to my success. It's hard to say what truly works and what doesn't. Cleaning up your act and your body and tracking your ovulation and having sex when you are ovulating is a good solid start.

We wanted to have another baby right away after my son was born but some outside circumstances but a damper on our plans. We weren't able to really decide what we wanted to do until he was a little over a year old. I was worried it was too late so I had blood work done and my doctor called me. BTW and FYI it's never good when the doctor calls. I will go into more detail later but know that when a nurse calls you are fine. When they have to upgrade you to speak with a doctor es no bueno. My doctor told me that my blood work indicated that I had pre-menopausal hormones rocking. I was put on Clomid for a few months. I did not like it and stopped using it. The debate in our house was how much intervention we should be willing to do. The phrase 'it's in God's hands' means different things to different people. Talk to a friend of mine and she will tell you God created the doctors who developed the fertility treatments so it's all good. My husband and I weren't willing to do any medical intervention. Taking a few months of an ovulation stimulating drug was enough for us. They made me angry, they made me moody, and made my periods so painful and awful. It was not for me. Lastly it moved my ovulation around. I was very precise and consistent. I had a lunar cycle with ovulation on day 11 or 12 at the latest. The two months while I was on Clomid and the subsequent few months after my ovulation shifted, it went up to day 10 and my monitor showed I was ovulating sometimes for 2-3 days in a row. There was a few month period where we thought that's it. That my body had finally succumbed to old age and more kids wasn't an option. I'm glad we persisted and kept trying. I'm thrilled that we gave it a true valiant effort and it paid off.

At 4,6 almost 47, my husband and I wish we still had a window that we felt safe about. We feel like we've rolled the dice too many times and we have to be smart and cash out at the casino. My risk factors are through the roof and at 44 his are creeping up there too. Six weeks post partum with my last baby I had the latest IUD implanted. Of course during the procedure I'm asking the doctor how reversible it is if we wanted to try for one more. We look at our beautiful wonderful amazing kids and wish we could go for another. However I digress so in sum, if you want to get pregnant clean up your act and have sex. Lots of it. It's fun and it's good for you. Enjoy yourself it's a celebration. Do your homework and talk to your doctor and find a philosophy and a school of thought you buy into and get Kenny Rodgers on that ass and know when to hold 'em and stick with it and know when to fold 'em and move onto another technique or practice. Sometimes your most scare resource not just your eggs but time. I suggesting finding out as soon as possible what your hormone levels look like. Nothing is a sure answer. No technique is a guarantee however being forewarned is forearmed and it is such a balance between gathering facts and information overload. Good luck and God speed. Enjoy yourself. The happier you are conceiving the happier you will be in general. Applying the old adage that what you are doing or feeling on New Years will set the tone for the rest of your year, be happy and have fun. It's sex and once it becomes work you are going down a bad path.

Again not having real fertility issues I'm by no means an expert but for the couples I've known who've had problems it's a divisive situation. As a woman, you are supposed to be built to have babies. Its part of your anatomical design. So what happens when you can't? It's very popular now days to choose not to. For everyone who does that it seems that there is a slurry of those who've chosen to have children but for some reason or another can't. I can tell you that there were a few months there where we were trying, not 100% perfectly but trying and it wasn't happening. Getting your period becomes this super depressing event. You've let everyone down, yourself and your husband and your family. We chose to have more children not just for ourselves but for our other kids. We saw how much they enjoyed their siblings and we wanted them to have another. So you've failed as a woman every month when your period comes. Everyone really does have a different experience and different road. Most couples I've ran into with fertility issues talk about how having sex becomes all about business. That the fun and joy is taken out of it. I recently read a quote that says sex is like pizza. Even bad pizza is still pizza. Right? I mean who are we kidding here. Sex is kind of fun no matter what. Syncing up the timing can be a bit time consuming, no pun intended, but its worth it. It's not that huge of a sacrifice to have to plan and calculate the timing out a few sessions of sex. I know some couples who've had a lot of luck again with just relaxing. After going full board with their baby making efforts and the testing and the hormone injections and the overall anxiety and intervention once they were able to take it down a notch, boom. Conception. One of my best friends had a terrible time getting and maintaining a pregnancy. Spent a small fortune on treatments and intervention. Then boom 3 months after her first was born she was pregnant without any extra efforts or hormones, the good old fashioned way.

Recently I had a neighbor come up to me telling me about an early term miscarriage she had last year and how they haven't used protection since and she doesn't understand why she isn't pregnant. She reeked of martinis and cigarettes. Do your self a favor and if you really want to get pregnant, live clean. No booze or cigarettes. You don't have to eat perfect but cut out some of the junk and take a prenatal vitamin daily. It's not that hard and they are changes you will have to make when you are pregnant anyway so why not start now so it's not such a shock to you when you have to. Far better to acclimate before hand then to slip or have a moment of weakness when you are pregnant. There is no room for that, especially if you are older and/or have had trouble. Just live clean. Track your ovulation and have sex a few days before and a few days after. Simple simple. So invest in the ClearBlue

Easy ovulation monitor. It's cheap compared to seeing a fertility specialists who are going to recommend you do it anyway. Now I've been told you can't give your monitor to anyone. That once you've used it its calibrated to you. I think that's a falsity put out there by ClearBlue Easy but that's me being old and jaded. Then you know you are serious to, cause who wants to waste that money. Where you can save some green is the prenatal vitamins. The target brand is $7 for 250 tablets. And they don't make you feel sick after you take them like some of the other very expensive ones. Pregnancy tests are cheap, you can get them at the 99 cent store if you want to buy them in bulk. Then I'll discuss in depth when we get into the medical stuff, the new MaterniT21 assay from Sequenom. Without insurance is $2200. With it's about $250. A full genetic profile just with a blood test on you around week 10. Do it. Don't even think about not doing it. It saved me from having an amnio and a lot of high risk appointments during my last pregnancy. Don't be cheap. Babies are way more expensive and you are saving on birth control anyway right? So start immediately. Prenatal vitamins can only help. I took them for 5 years straight, missed a few days here and there but yup 5 years. I monitored my periods and ovulation religiously for 4 years. Once you get the routine going it becomes second nature. By the time you discover a fertility problem it may be too late, expensive or time consuming to try and resolve it.

We should all be so grateful to the power of the celebrity that has made being pregnant in vogue as well as opened our eyes to so many alternatives and making them acceptable like adoption and surrogacy. The spotlight also focuses on celebrity couples who are together for a short time and end up pregnant. I'm sure every time a fertility challenged couple reads about someone like Rob Kardashian and his girlfriend Blac Chyna expecting a baby after dating only a few months thinks damn, well at least they have the money to care for it but there are a million stories like that out there. Very few couples are like us older ladies in that we are well planned out and calculated. For the vast majority of especially younger couples it is an accident or a surprise. Let me tell you, I wanted to get pregnant. I put the time and energy and planning in and got pregnant. There was no OOOPPS to any of it. I was thankful and I was elated and I was blessed and I was happy but I wasn't surprised. It used to be you would speak about adopted children in a manner that you knew they were really really wanted. Someone fought hard and went through a lot of usually very difficult red tape to have that child be a part of their family. Older moms can look upon their children in a similar light. If you are having one or a whole bunch this late in your fertility window it's all good and every one is a miracle. When I'm coherent and awake enough on most days I look at my children in awe. As I'm putting out fires and handling crisis's and managing the chaos I catch myself staring at little hands and little toes and thanking god above for gifting me with these treasures. It doesn't make it any easier. But it's all so worth it. All of the sacrifice and hardship is gone and all you have are beautiful little people staring back at you. Climbing on you. Pulling your hair. Getting you dirty with their ketchup and sugar covered hands. You are smart. Once you figure out your cycle and your timings you can greatly increase your chances of conceiving if that's what your body is capable of, by being smart and hitting that with the Jericho missile when you only want a weapon you only have to fire once.

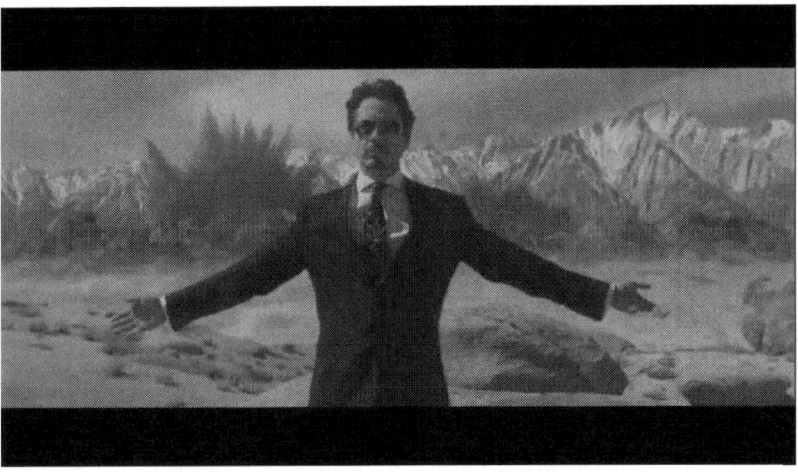

Movie "Iron Man" Marvel Entertainment 2008

That's how dad did it. That's how America does it. And it's worked out pretty well so far. Blast that egg with everything you've got.

Speaking of dad, it goes without say to make sure you partner is on board. These are not things to undertake alone. There is a pivotal scene in the movie Juno where Justin Bateman (the husband) tells Jennifer Garner (the adoptive wife) that he isn't ready yet. It all happened too fast. Don't be like them. Make sure your partner is on board and you aren't working your ovulation dates behind their backs and liquoring them up on the right night so you can conceive. I never understood women who get pregnant "on accident" or to try and manipulate a person or a situation. All of this will be hard enough so don't alienate your partner before you even begin and make sure they are on board first. If after a discussion they say they aren't ready and you are already over 40 then your relationship needs to be readdressed. Hoping that they will come around when you turn up pregnant is not realistic. If you think your partner is that much of an asshole and doesn't want to have a baby, then that seems to be a big giant red flag. If you think your partner is too stupid to know what they want and you can manipulate the situation, again doesn't seem like a healthy relationship to start a family in. Everyone deserves respect and honesty. This is a long and tough road and you need support, not animosity to walk down it.

Finally, it's the beginning of the end. For those of you that don't know the over the counter pregnancy tests are ridiculously accurate, right. You don't need to buy the $20 one at the CVS, the ones at the 99 cent store work just as well, without some of the fancy display features, but just as well. The test simply detects a hormone in your system that is present when you are pregnant. No magic. If you are like me and want to take several tests, before the beginning of each period while you are pregnant. I've probably taken 50 tests, including one recently thinking that the birth control implant I have wasn't working properly. I even saved the positive ones from my first and second pregnancies. Yeah all of that gross saving of things wears off at some point, thank God. Foreskin, umm no thanks. Belly button, nope not for me. If you don't know when you are pregnant, I'm not sure I can help you. I didn't have an accidental pregnancies. I was anxiously anticipating a positive pregnancy test or my period every month. There wasn't any well I don't know I might be late, I'm not sure. No I knew all of the dates, timings, when I should and shouldn't be having my period, ovulating, or even implanting an egg. Not a lot of guess work here. Some cold hard date calculating and running different ovulation apps.

I became at expert at the physiological events between ovulation to fertilization to implantation. I knew what was happening when, along with help from my apps. It takes a few days from ovulation, to fertilization, for the egg to drop and finally implant in your uterine lining. That's when the magic happens. I found myself taking it easy on those days, no jumping no hiking, but then again you aren't that fragile and your body systems aren't that easy to disrupt. Looking back I've heard tons of stories from women who didn't know they were pregnant yet and they were drinking Saki at an all you can eat sushi bar. I myself went hiking and to the trampoline park on implantation week before I knew I was pregnant with my daughter. Worked out fine for me, no problems. So you have that stick in your hand that says yes you are pregnant, what is the nest step? Maybe even more than one stick. Possibly a baker's dozen. I averaged 2-4 the months I wasn't pregnant, just to be sure over a few different days, starting a few days before my period was due until I got it. For those lucky moments, I took 6-8. You know, just to be sure. I saved them for a while. Yuck. Just to look at. So gross. It wasn't like I was going to put it in their baby scrap books so I don't know what I was thinking. After you confirm you are pregnant you call your doctor. They ask if you've had a test. You say yes. If you say no they send you to the lab for a blood draw. I did that with my first pregnancy to confirm. Waste of time and money but if you need that reassurance knock yourself out. Then you schedule your first appointment. The amazing start of your adventure, for every journey of 1000 miles begins with a single step, which is in this case is the 8 week visit.

4. Confused Ladies And Calling Your Doctor. C'me On Man!

I'm not a doctor. No shit. I don't have a doctor contributing to this book. Really? If you have any questions what so ever while you are pregnant, before you are pregnant, after you are pregnant, **CALL YOUR DOCTOR.** Don't be a douche bag and don't put the life of your child in jeopardy by either taking your medical advice from a book or a blog or by not having the courage to call. There usually is someone available to speak with you 24 hours a day. Now yes there are such thing as a dumb question but being pregnant gives you a free pass. There are so many things you don't know. So many things I didn't know. I can't tell you how many times I found myself surprised by something that happened with my body or my baby. Even with the entire internet at my disposal, WebMD, blogs, books I still got caught off guard. So call. Any day. Any time. If you are concerned enough about something that is going on then it's serious enough to call and get an answer for. That's what you are paying for if you think about it. The average pregnancy bills out at over $20,000. A high risk one like the ones I had cost more, and if you put fertility treatments and a c-section in the mix is the cherry on the top and run you the cost of a car if not a small house. I had different insurances for different pregnancies. Some had higher premiums and lower out of pocket maximums. That worked out well while I was pregnant the last time as it helped me manage my monthly cash flow better. With my son I had tons of appointments as I was mega high risk. I had insurance with a lower premium and a higher deductible. That was a bit of a sting as the costs were decent plus the hospital fees were pretty steep. It's no fun seeing a big bill when you are at home freaking out with a new baby. My bills without insurance adjustment for just the hospital totaled well over $25,000 for a vaginal delivery with no complications and 48 hour stay. Either way for all of the money you put out you have more than paid for ANY phone call you might make. 3am, trust me there is someone on call at the local hospital who can answer your question. Babies don't usually come during the 9am-5pm Monday through Friday shift and neither do issues or questions about your pregnancy. Call. If it's something simple usually your doctor's nurse can answer it. More complicated issues will be directed to an MD on call. The people who work in my doctor's office who answer the phones and do the scheduling are very knowledgeable and are excellent dispatchers to insure that calls are answered by the right person. Just call. Don't read some idiot's blog to try and get an answer to something that is bothering you or worse yet scaring you at 4 o'clock in the morning. Just call and get a doctor's word for it. There is so much misinformation out there, just call and get a real medical answer. It's worth it's weight in peace of mind. Having said that be prepared for the answer. With malpractice suits and all of the other variables that effect how doctor's can administer care now a days most medical professionals are in cover their ass mode to reduce their personal and professional liability. If you feel like you are having contractions you are going to be told to go to nearest hospital for monitoring. If you are bleeding you are going to be told to monitor the output and go in if it exceeds a critical amount, which is like one pad in a few hours worth btw. However if you have heartburn, a fever, or anything pretty mild you will be told what medications you can and can't take and have your concern addressed. "Oh yeah, that's perfectly normal," direct quote by Dr. R. Salzetti said to me about a million times. Just call. You paid for it, you earned it and even the most informed person in the world doesn't have the answers for everything so call a medical professional.

I can't tell you again how many really ill-informed not very bright folks who probably don't have jobs (do the reasoning on that one) sit around all day on the pregnancy blogs and respond when you post a question or issue. It's not pretty. I remember distinctly being appalled by the take a bunch of folks had on a pregnancy app community I frequented regarding TDAP vaccines. This is the tetanus, pertussis, etc. vaccine and its recommended for not only mommies but all adult care givers since the baby can't have one right away and is highly susceptible especially to pertussis, which is whooping cough. At the time there was an outbreak in California and I live in San Diego which based on its proximity to Mexico made us especially vulnerable since at the time the Mexican government didn't require whooping cough vaccines and it was thought that the lax vaccine standards in Mexico made the border populations much more vulnerable to things like whooping cough and tuberculosis. The trolls on this site came back with everything from it's all false propaganda by the pharmaceutical companies to there is no proof it saves lives by getting vaccinated. These are the types of people who take the time energy and effort to monitor and respond on web based open communities, where opinions are like assholes, you know the rest. Not people like me who work and who are educated and would never leave a critical decision like getting vaccinated up to the opinions of people on a web site community forum. Do you care more about your child's life and well being than bothering someone at 2am with a phone call and potentially inconveniencing them or looking foolish by asking a stupid question? You should care more about your baby and if you don't now it the time to realign your values and thinking. Speaking of not calling your doctor when you should, don't be embarrassed if you feel you call too much. Yes they are going to talk about you. Yes you may end up being the talk around the lounge the next day when the nurses are getting a snack but what do you care. You will probably be talked about anyway. The problem we all have is not only do we not know anything we have no idea the absolute abyss of what we don't know. For many of us this is our first and only. For us older ladies we have fought so hard to be here, yes we are going to call with every issue now and wait until we start dealing with our pediatricians. Even if we have a sister with a ton of kids or a mom who raised a whole slew with no help it's not the same to get advice or information from them than it is to get it from an MD.

In sharp contrast, I also never walked into a doctor's office and thought, this person knows everything, I'm going to trust them implicitly, follow everything they tell me and trust that they will always keep me 100% informed and have all of the right answers. Doctor's are educated and experienced but no one should blindly earn your trust. Again another lesson in parenting, you have to be an advocate for you and yours. I adore my doctor, but I always did independent research. I did not for a second not realize that by gaining weight I could adversely effect my blood pressure and sugar levels. I knew that I was at a crazy high risk for all types of complications not only to the baby but to my health. You are the explorer on this journey with the doctor and nurses as your guides but you bear the responsibility for your decisions. I have friends like myself in high risk categories who after their first high risk pregnancy and all of the doctoring and testing that's involved opted out of all testing, with the assumption if something is wrong I will deal with it. Now I have other friends who say be prepared. I understand both points of view. The doctoring is excessive and it's very hard on anyone, not only you and your stress levels but on your spouse. There were a few appointments my husband couldn't make and I wished he had been there for sure. Its just tough from the get go. Your doctor is a guide, not a god and from a pragmatic point of view your doctor's nurse is one of your best resources. I also had great advice from my yoga instructor so I felt that like covered both spectrums. Medical and kind of error on the side of caution with holistic practices from my yoga instructor and going with the flow. I tended to have my philosophies more in the middle.

5. Who's House? Run's House. Paging Dr. 'Cover Yo Ass.'

Having told you to call your doctor with questions also keep in mind that your medical care can be dictated by you. Of course you should follow the doctor's recommendations for testing and screenings, appointments, diets and what to do and what not to do. I can tell you after 3 pregnancies I haven't met a single person who does NOT eat something from the do not eat list. Everyone indulges in something whether it's sushi or lunchmeat or hotdogs or cantaloupe. Exercise caution and care and it's good to know all of the things you aren't supposed to do but keep in mind that is a list of questionable practices that may or may not have any bearing on your health or the health of your unborn child. I can tell you what I did. I didn't eat sushi because that just seemed like asking for trouble. I colored my hair. Oh my stars. Yes more than once, with a box at home and even in a salon. I had my toes done. I had massages. Now with both of those you need to tell the therapist / technician that you are pregnant if they look at you with a blank stare take a pass and leave. For nails they are not supposed to overly rub your calves, and for massages positioning is key along with an additional pillow so you are not on your belly, duh but not. I ate hot dogs more than once and lunchmeat. There is a restriction on doing abdominal exercises, laying on your back, etc. I didn't do sit ups – that was SO not a problem.

I did try to take over the direction of my medical care on my last pregnancy. I was tired of having appointments every 3 weeks because of my very high risk status. For my first two pregnancies I did everything that was recommended to do with regards to doctor's appointments, tests and screenings. I sat down early with my primary OB and perinatalogist during my last pregnancy and let them know I wasn't game for all of that doctoring again. First having to find a sitter for a toddler for appointments every few weeks is a drag. The worst part of that pregnancy for me was the last month when the appointments escalated and I couldn't talk myself out of the twice a week appointments for the last 3 weeks. Yuck. Hated it. But you are seriously in charge of some of the direction. You can consult with the doctor about what you feel comfortable with. I have friends who were in high risk categories who had very minimal monitoring. As it turned out it kind of backfired on them, there is that fine line between all of this technology is available so you can see and hear your baby quite often. You can go to the 4D ultrasound place and gets frameable snapshots made. One of my friends husband was obsessed with the 4D ultrasound and they went all of the time and even has the postage stamps for her shower invites as a picture of this baby in the womb. Not my style but that is available. You can even buy an at home Doppler so you can hear your little one. Keep in mind there is also the philosophy that the doctor and their group is doing everything possible to cover their ass. That you, even as a unique being with a unique pregnancy, has been placed on a very generic outlined plan of care depending on your age and status. The plan that mitigates and limits their liability the most. It's hard.

Going through a high risk pregnancy, let alone 3 in a row, takes it toll on you mentally. Being older and putting your body through the hormones and weight gains and loses and all of the other physical side effects is one thing, but the emotional stress of carrying a child coupled with the impending doom of being older and the potential short and long term risks to you and the baby are insane. It doesn't stop. The negativity. The statistics. The percentages. After you are in the clear with the baby and you feel like you can let up and take a breath and relax for a moment, the bastards start it with the risks to you like preeclampsia and gestational diabetes. They are always coming at you with a negative spin if you are older. It does not let up even for a day. The fear and anxiety and near panic are constant and perpetually fueled by your doctor, by reading on line posts and chats, and of course your own sick mind hopped up on hormones and donuts and taking your places that the most horrific movie wouldn't even dare go. The Human Caterpillar has nothing on you, your mind will take you dark obsessive places. Fear and raging hormones will lead you down a path that a lot of women have a hard time escaping. A panicked reel of possible tragedies played in super fast speed on the screen in your head. I had blurbs I read imprinted and replaying on a loop especially during restless nights when I was stressed trying to get my kick count so I didn't have to go down to the hospital for monitoring and so uncomfortable that I couldn't sleep. There are a quite a few children on our street who are challenged with Autism, and I see their families work so hard to cope and keep things together that are absolutely bursting as the seams. It becomes terrifying when you realize your odds of having some type of developmental disorder as a late in life mom that is mind blowingly large and that's terrifying. So you have both your imagined and real fear, which is fun, right? Especially having said that keep in mind that being pregnant at this age requires you to be an active participant. You have to read and be an informed advocate for yourself and your baby. You have to sort out the real versus the fictional pressing issues and make a list for your doctor to address during your visits, or take the time each week and call your doctor's nurse. You might think you are being a pain in the ass. It's mentally, physically and emotionally exhausting. But, if you are only going to get one shot at this do it right will ya.

You own it, you better never let it go
You only get one shot, do not miss your chance to blow
This opportunity comes once in a lifetime

It is your job to recognize that the doctor is a resource and you have to do your own independent research in order to make this work for you. It's overwhelming but for some of us this is it, there won't be another chance so you have to put everything you have into it. It's hard. It's scary. Suck it up. You go for an ultrasound and instead of going in a room where someone tells you everything looks great you have the perinatalogist on call counseling you about all of your odds of Down's Syndrome and how you don't have this marker or that one but there is a blur on the images and you might have that one. I had ultrasounds where the technician wouldn't tell us anything. We had to have a consultation afterwards. What a joy that was. Complete doom as the doctor who you may or not ever see again reads your chart and goes over all of the factors that stand out to them, primarily your age and any previous history of loss or problems which is such a treat and joy in an of it's self then they start going over the potential issues with your current baby. I can't tell you how fun it is to relive the heartbreak of a loss, in detail, sitting in a tarp made out of paper towels with your butt sweat sticking you to the exam table talking with a medical provider who, as mentioned, you more than likely are never going encounter again, all because they are curious about an anomaly on your chart and want to reduce their liability. I once had a nurse taking my weight and blood pressure and asking for a urine sample while I was a few months pregnant with my son and she referenced the loss on my chart and really started interrogating me about it. I was less than 6 months removed from delivering a dead baby and she wanted to know all about it. Absolute misery. I would walk away from those sessions needing not only a real long nap because I was just exhausted by it but I'd be in a funk for at least a day going over the data and what was said and what was implied, over and over again in my head.

While pregnant with my son and being as high risk as you could be after having a loss right before this pregnancy, it just never stopped. After my anatomical ultrasound around week 17 I was counseling by a one hit wonder, perinatalogist on call that the technician had found 4 of the multiple down's syndrome markers on that ultrasound. There were 'bright' spots on the heart and some other indicators. I also have a positive result on my first trimester screening. So how do I deal with this. This was the 2nd pregnancy I had, but the first time I had a positive trimester screening PLUS a potentially problematic ultrasound. Those words were booming in my head when I heard Down's Syndrome markers and the dark cloud of doom set over me, adding additional weight to the shoulders that were already bearing that recent loss. I was petrified. For better or for worse, I was also ready. Ready to make what would the hardest decision of my life. I could handle some special needs, but I know myself and in my heart of hearts even with a previous loss I would think twice about keeping a baby that had devastating problems and I could very well terminate the pregnancy. I'm a monster. I know. I also thought I knew that I didn't want to do it. I have friends with kids that are Autistic and the amount of extra work it takes verses a quasi normal child is off the charts. So what to do? I had an amnio scheduled in a few weeks. If that came back bad its almost right at the 20 week mark so if you want to terminate your pregnancy you have to do it fast or else have it done by someone who will perform a semi-illegal abortion. How was I to know for sure if the baby had a problem? Some problems are more obvious than others. Things missing like the top of the skull are easy to see, a genetic abnormality is a whole other ball of wax. I've heard horror stories of couples being told there is something wrong with their child then they decide to keep the pregnancy and prepare and hope for the best and the child turns out fine. So how do you know? How many experts and other opinions can you get, and how long before alternate blood work is done and results can be read? Not within the 20 weeks I speculate. What do you do? I knew I couldn't do special needs but I also knew I if it came to that I would have to go to extraordinary lengths to insure that there was something wrong. I thought in my mind I would probably have to travel to Los Angeles and have a whole battery of tests done. How can you be sure? Put cameras in there like they do for bypass surgery? Take a spinal tap off the embryo?

It wasn't until the amnio results came back and I was genetically in the clear did I take a deep breath. That was a very long 4 weeks from the time I was told there were issues, having the amnio, which is not a fun procedure, and then waiting for those results. And of course all of the negative counseling is in person, you are in an office, trapped, with statistics being thrown at you and you are exhausted from being pregnant and having traveled down to whatever hospital has an ultra high resolution ultrasound and it's a long, tiring appointment and a long day then to have some ass clown with an MD next to his name that you won't see again tell you about a spot on the heart or a blur on an image, some bullshit that what they aren't telling you is it's probably nothing and could be an error in the technique of the technician or just a manifestation of the positioning or movement on the baby so the tech didn't get a very clear picture. They don't tell you that part. They tell you your odds of down's at 1 in 2 and show you some rapidly rising chart mapping your age and risk assessment. Yikes.

Now when everything is fine they usually call you. Sometimes they don't and send a letter instead, requiring you to advocate for yourself to get test results as soon as they are available. I had about 4 ultrasounds where the tech won't talk to you, all analysis and interpretation had to be given by the doctor. A delay you have to factor in because the doctor has to take the time to review the images and look at your chart. I've had ultrasounds where the techs do talk to you and you can tell by their tone and how they chose their words if there is an issue or not. There are a few different levels of communication. With most high stakes test results come with a phone call and you usually talk to a nurse when everything is fine. When the doctor calls it's because something has come back questionable or bad and when the doctor calls and leaves you a message to call him back right away, that's when panic rightfully sets in. When they want to really scare you it's face to face. Finally be warned there are also random results that come in letter form in the mail. Feel free to call for a consult after you open those so you can actually understand what they mean. Go figure. That takes its toll too. The up and down and back and forth. Worse than a slapped together carnival ride where you fear for your life at every turn that the operator of the guys who assembled it forgot that critical bolt that holds it together or were drunk at 2am when they put it last night in the empty lot down the street from your house. I had to be prepared. I didn't want to think about it but I had to. If I was going to have all of the testing and know all of the issues before hand what was I willing to do. Was I willing to end the pregnancy if I found out we had a serious problem? How would I deal with that? What if the tests were flawed? Some of them are. The trimester screenings all factor your age into the results so if you are older you will test positive because it's weighted for age. WTF? That's one of those fun tests that isn't covered by insurance either, it's state regulated in California. It's overwhelming, exhausting and stress inducing. What is the alternative? It's not pretty to think about. The alternative is to say I won't do any of this testing and take my chances. Now a days with so many ways to know, could you go through a pregnancy not knowing? I wish I could have had the opportunity to consider it as well as had the opportunity to not have to have my baby at a hospital and try a birthing center as I wish everyone around me had been able to keep a secret and I hadn't found out the gender of my babies. As a grown up your wish list is based on a romantic image in your head. It isn't real and it isn't always practical. This isn't the place or time in your life to being taking risks. What you are doing is already risky enough. Now I agreed to donate a small sample of the fluid from my first amnio towards work on the test that became the MaterniT21. It makes you wonder with all of the tests and experiments if anyone has ever studied how the stress of having a late in life pregnancy effects the pregnancy and your child's brain chemistry. Especially with the tests that come out positive no matter what if you are older, now those are hardly what I would consider to be scientific. Pregnancy is magical, it's beautiful and even with some negative physical consequences I love it and wish I could be pregnant again. Now that's romantic and nostalgic and far away but while I was in it I was all business and it kind of has to be that way because there are some nasty cold hard truths staring at your from the other side of that clipboard. Do you want to know? If you don't and you can live with all of the consequences including that there may be something wrong that you could fix, then don't find out and I love you and support you in that. Me, I gotta know especially since it was business, it was a job, and I wanted to do my best.

A note about other medical professionals like dentists, optometrists, massage therapists, etc. Please remember you have to advocate your rights over your body and your unborn child. Do NOT take for granted that just because someone is a doctor or therapist that they have any working knowledge or understanding of how to treat you and what not to do to you while you are pregnant or might be pregnant. With regards to dentists, opt OUT of dental x-rays, anesthesia, gas, Novocain, etc. You will live and can get your fillings done after your pregnancy. They don't know, just because they are also doctors don't think for a minute they understand what trying to get and being pregnant means and how it should effect your course of treatment. It's a hard lesson to learn and I've had to learn it more than once with a slew of different so called professionals pushing me to do x-rays and other non urgent testing just to rack up their billable procedures.

The Eye Doctor. My eyes went screwy. Really screwy. According to my eye doctor my stigmatisms were altered while pregnant because the shape of your eye can change. This coupled with being older and pre-menopausal really put the hex on my eye sight. I went from being someone who was totally corrected by contacts and could see very well with my glasses to having contacts prescribed to me that were very different before and after various pregnancies. My favorite eye appointment was a few months into my first pregnancy. It was an annual appointment to get a years worth of contacts. The doctor kept remarking that my prescription had really changed. I told him 6-8 times that I was pregnant. He didn't listen, just kept remarking as he was writing down the results of my exam that my eyes had really changed. I kept repeating that I was pregnant. It was a Saturday and this ass bag was cranky and annoyed to begin with. Finally he looked at me instead of the chart and said pregnant, oh well come back when you aren't. Little did he know I would go on to lose that baby a few months later and his words would resonate for years to come. I also had to live with my new prescription from him that was much higher than my old one for the next year. I was blessed enough to get pregnant again and I bypassed that year's exam because I was wearing my glasses more and not blowing through my lenses at a regular rate and my eyes were shifting again. After my son was born I went back in because I really couldn't see. I was getting headaches and my vision was blurry and it made me really irritable. I thought it was the sleep deprivation or the exhaustion.

Turns out the next ophthalmologist I saw was also a new mom and she explained to me that I had been given a prescription that was too strong and, as mentioned above, that your eyes can really change while you are pregnant. She changed me back to a lower correction and I was good until the next pregnancy. After my daughter was born my glasses weren't working for me anymore. I couldn't read text and I could not see at dusk at all which made me scared to drive. My contacts were ok except I couldn't read fine print on anything and I'd had to put things into natural light to really get a good look at it. My glasses weren't working for me at all. The new eye doctor found that I now had dry eye, a premenopausal and age related development and that I required bifocals as my eyes had shifted and in addition to being near sighted I had become far sighted as well. The stigmatism I already had that has reshaped my eyeball after all of the pregnancies and hormonal ups and downs into something similar to deflate-a-gate. I need reading glasses and the harsh reality is that I'm no longer a decent candidate for laser correction because of all of my issues. Well isn't that super. So I'm old but I'm a new mom so I'm having all of those symptoms playing out in additional to be totally exhausted and scatter brained. My grandfather got really cranky as he was getting older. His hearing, eyesight and memory started going and it made him just nasty mean. Admittedly I feel the same way some days. I'm so tired my brain doesn't fire right and my eyes and hearing are shot.

Dentist. Another fun side effect I had was bleeding gums. Oh my dentist had a field day with me. I developed these gums that if you touched them they bled. I'm no slouch in the dental hygiene department. At minimum I went to the dentist 2-3 times a year. I brush with a sonic brush 2-4 times a day and my gum care was educated and pretty good, but not always regular. This earned me a ration of grief from dental hygienists. Please please remember that in everything that happens to you – you DO have a say. I have one major major regret going to the dentist while pregnant. I didn't know I was pregnant but I knew I was trying and one of the ways the dentist makes money is to charge your insurance for x-rays every year and every time I went the hygienist would really pressure me into getting them. I used to say oh next time, next time. Well I caved in one visit, again not knowing I was pregnant, because I hadn't had them in a while. I regret that terribly. I lost that baby and having those x-rays is one of only a few miniscule things I did wrong during that pregnancy that had the slightest chance of having caused the defect and or issue that resulted in her not making it. Anyway for the next few years I told them to crew off when they told me I had to get x-rays. It became an uncomfortable fight that made me opt out of going to the dentist all together. I'm actually stuck right now trying to find a new dentist. My insurance changed and no one will see me with out an initial exam and x-rays and I can't afford to go back to my old dentist without insurance, though I'm really considering it just to get my teeth cleaned. I'm still nursing and I want no part of any hulk level radiation thank you. I tell them I'm pregnant, or trying to get pregnant and don't know yet. That should get them off your back, but not always. Anyway while pregnant some women develop a condition by which your gums bled when you touch them. Not to mention gushed like a slasher movie when the hygienist came after them with sonic irradiated metal picks. Something about being pregnant too the sonic dental picks gave me a total migraine. I was diligent about getting my teeth cleaned but it was torture. To this day my gums are still screwy and in conjunction with gorging myself on sweets while knocked up I have a handful of small cavities. I do my best with an ultrasonic toothbrush and the waterpik. After finally caving in recently and getting myself down to a dentist I found they wouldn't clean my teeth without x-rays. A frustrating waste of an hour for sure. I am still nursing and refuse the exposure. So my teeth will suffer. This alleged dentist I just recently went to see also before looking in my mouth said he was going to screen me for head and neck cancers and told me after being the chair for 30 seconds that he thought I had a thyroid tumor. He also said without x-rays that I had 3 cavities and I could come back next time for fillings and maybe a cleaning then. Total load of bullshit. I told them I thought I was pregnant and that's why I didn't want x-rays, I had called earlier to make an appointment and told them I wanted to pass on x-rays because I was nursing and the appointment booker was arguing with me about the safety of x-rays. I didn't want an argument so I said I might be pregnant and the doctor was all pissy and proceeded to tell me he thought I had thyroid cancer. Because there is nothing like adding to the stress of a potentially pregnant 47 year old woman by telling her you think, without an oncology degree or an MD, that someone has cancer. There are negligent and bad doctors out there. They are everywhere.

My point is that just because someone is a medical professional, even an OB, doesn't make them a good person or even a knowledgeable person. They aren't to be completely revered and trusted. Educate yourself. You have to be your own boss, your own champion and your own defender.

II. Pregnant? Now What?

6. McSteamy, Nurse Ratchet And Dealing With Insurance.

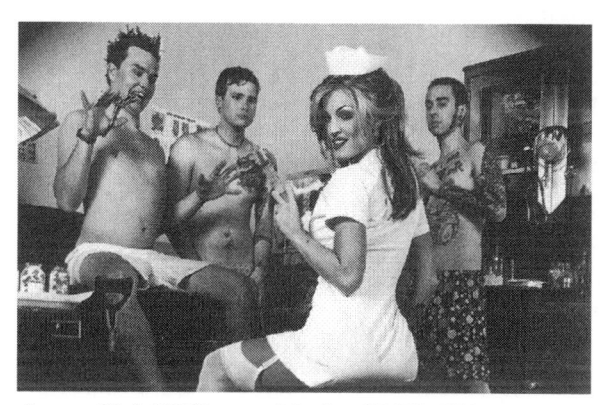

Source: Blink 182 "Enema of the State" MCA 1999

You can have a McSteamy or a McDreamy. I've seen so many doctors and medical professionals over the past few years it makes me dizzy. Over 2 dozen different nurses and about the same amount of ultrasound technicians. Half a dozen pediatricians, phlebotomists, several perinatalogists and a handful of OBs. I estimate over 100 medical personnel over the past few years. I've had some great looking doctors, George Clooney in ER good looking. I've had some doctors I would absolutely put my life in their hands and trust their judgment implicitly. My regular OB and current pediatrician are the top two of those. Unfortunately I've also had some eeehhh not so much, just covering their ass doctors. A few my husband wanted to punch because they were so cold and callus just reading off statistics about how doomed our pregnancy was. I've had doctors who I only saw once who just seemed lost and stuck in liability reduction mode and it caused a negative ripple in my pregnancy.

Imagine having a relationship with someone that is more intimate with anyone else on the planet other than your husband or partner. If you have a baby solo, which is awesome especially given some of the husbands and partners I encounter that are real assholes, then that person literally has his or her hands in you probably more than anyone. This is someone who is tracking all of your biological statistics. Someone who sees you at your worst. Trust in this relationship is paramount as he or she is your guide in a very complicated and treacherous journey.

So here were are at the beginning of the next phase holding a positive pregnancy test. Let me tell you having a baby is so super expensive. **Before you go for your first appointment call your insurance company.** This becomes very difficult as you are about to hit a crossroads and your first dilemma. Finding your regular OB. Do you already have one? Great. If not it can get sticky and tricky. I did not. As someone who was never ill, I would have my yearly women wellness check done by my primary doctor. Now I did know what my coverage was in regards to the fact that the clinic I went to see my GP at was part of the" in network" group. These are terms you need to familiarize yourself with immediately. In network to me means that the facility and or doctor is covered under the principal umbrella of your insurance. Out of network are facilities and doctors outside of that primary coverage. You can always call the billing for a certain facility and tell them your coverage and they will let you know if they accept it. Usually if the facility and or clinic accept your coverage, you can assume all of the doctors there do as well. In my case I go to Scripps clinic. A huge network of several facility and hospitals which were all covered under the larger umbrella of my coverage. Each baby still cost me about $10,000 out of pocket and that was with high end PPO coverage. At the particular location I go they had several OB's on staff to and I literally chose the one that had the first availably to see me at the 8 week point. Not everyone is so lucky nor wants to do things so blindly. Your first appointment isn't so critical, so you want to start fine tuning the OB group you want to be in and the doctor you want to see regularly. Friends, relatives, co-workers can all give you a recommendations, just call first to make sure they take your coverage. What you may want to do is prepare a list of questions for your first appointment as most doctors are completely prepared for this. They expect you to be very nervous, cautious, wary, scared, and inquisitive. You can ask a million questions but the meat of the matter is the questions you don't even know to ask yet. Truly you want to find someone who fits well with your personality because you will be spending a lot of time together. That person gets a real view not only of your body but of your life, your marriage, your highs and lows, your fears, your ever growing ass and all of that. You want to find someone you feel comfortable talking about changes that are happening to you body about, from gas to a smelly crotch, from pain during sex to heartburn. These are not light topics. You are in a perpetual state of embarrassment with whomever you chose. So chose wisely. Try a few. They shouldn't take offense if you chose not to stay with them and if someone does, then they weren't the right match for you anyway.

As in my case, it's sometimes the luck of the draw. Remember that you will also start to get very emotional so any issues like feeling your doctor doesn't listen to you, or isn't helping or addressing your problems or concerns will be magnified. If I could do it again I would ask the following: What are you going to tell me? Are you going to tell me everything? Every remote possibility of a rare or obscure issue? Is your approach aggressive or more wait and see? There are some very critical time frames for late in life pregnancies, the most important is between having an amniocentesis and the time you have to legally terminate your pregnancy. It's about 2 weeks. You have to be sure and be ready to make some very difficult decisions and you need someone who can effectively guide you.

As vital as the doctor is, and there you initially have a choice in which you see, the medical staff you end up dealing with the most are the nurses. I've had nurses who looked pissed off to be dealing with me. Nurses who seemed lost. Nurses who made me cry. One nurse who was my hero. She sat and held my hand during one of my darkest days and she was more than part of my medical care, she was my friend and a true care giver. Kathy is always in my heart for her kindness and compassion waiting with me in the ultrasound area, while my emergency scan was ordered and performed and I learned we had lost our first baby. I make a point to try and see her every time I'm at the same medical center. When we visit the pediatrician we do our best to stop by as rarely does your OB and their team get to actually see the results of their efforts. She's one of those people who is in the right profession, she is on point and does her job impeccably. She was my friend, my cheerleader, always with a smile and support. I had another nurse who took a very scared woman ready to give birth who had not attended or really paid much mind to natural child birth techniques and guided me through an unexpected drug free delivery with flying colors all the while telling me how great a job I was doing which made me kind of want to tell her to shut up but she was so sweet and calm and got me on point. Thank you and shout out to Danielle. My nurse and last minute drug free birth coach as my husband and I had arrogantly glossed over that possibility.

Keep a spreadsheet of your appointments, receipts of any payments, and organize all of the statements and claim forms that you will be amassing over the next year. You will be getting bills months later that say now due or overdue. Managing the financial aspect of your care is stressful and time consuming so don't just shove all of the claims and billing statements in a drawer to sort out later. Deal with them on a regular basis to stay on top of them.

Both of the insurance coverages we had during my pregnancies assigned a nurse to call and talk to me about things are going and to track my progress. Part of this is very savvy on their part. They want to collect data on you for their risk analysis so they can figure out how to raise, oh sorry 'adjust,' premiums in the future. Its comforting to have another medical professional assigned to you, kind of like a case worker on behalf of your insurance. I didn't use the service so I don't know how helpful they are. I found that my doctor's nurse and the women who did the scheduling in the OB office I went to were very proficient in dealing with insurance, covered procedures, what needed advance authority, etc.

Most of my regular check ups were the same. My husband would b.s. with the doctor about the latest happenings in college football while I was on the exam table. Ob's in general have the gift of gab to try and put you at ease and distract you from what they are doing. I came to realize after going to that doctor for 4 years straight that my husband and I were kind of unique. Usually he saw women alone, even the pregnant ones, and mostly older responsible ones getting their yearly exams. When the husbands did show up they were usually in a suit on a break from work. The husbands I saw always looked like fish out of water. My husband on the other hand was very relaxed and going with the flow. He is very social and great at making small talk which cuts out so much of the tension of being at the doctor. After chatting it up with my husband the doctor would look at my stats, blood pressure mostly and weight. He would tell me what to expect next appointment whether it was an ultrasound or screening or just a regular check up. Most of my appointments consisted of me having no questions or concerns. Sometimes, however I would unload depending on my mood and hit him with half a dozen complaints at once. Almost always written off as 'completely normal' and we would move on. I can actually see his face and hear his voice as I'm recanting this. He would kind of close his eyes and shake his head slightly as to dismiss my concern all together and assure me, 'perfectly normal.' Nothing to be alarmed about. Like when your kid falls down and hurts themselves and they are screaming bloody murder and you say, oh you are fine, let's go. It keeps the anxiety or the hysteria from building by diffusing the panic. My doctor was my friend and his temperament was perfect for me at my stage of life. Might not work for everyone but almost anyone I ever met when I told them he was my doctor looked at me in awe and told me how lucky I was. Yes I was and I hit the jackpot across the board. Our temperaments matched, my husband loved him, his nurse was one of the most wonderful fairy godmother ladies in my life during this journey, #WINNING across the board. Tiger's blood.

7. Take Off All Of Your Clothes And Put On This Paper Towel.

I can give you an overview of 3 different pregnancies and the different doctors appointments for each. Double check and check your insurance again. If you have coverage with a deductible you are going to hit that real fast, maybe on the first visit even. Most laboratory work is either covered as a percentage and some isn't covered at all. Most appointments and routine testing like ultrasounds etc. are covered. None of my monthly appointments required a co-pay but almost all of my lab work was paid on the % covered basis, so 80% up to $10,000 out of pocket for the calendar year.

You take a pregnancy test, maybe even a few days before your period is due and it comes up positive!!! JOY! Then you take a few more to confirm and call to make that first appointment which you are told won't happen until you've hit that critical 8 week mark.

Appointments everyone has:
8 week initial appointment. Your first ultrasound and confirmation of viability and pregnancy. An internal ultrasound so a giant rod is inserted into your whoo haa. Fun. Your first taste of plastic gloves and tons of lube. These are usually done in office, some doctors have a special ultrasound room and the resolution is pretty basic. You will see an alien like form in your uterus and hear and hopefully see a heartbeat. Also a full OB exam with smears and swabs to identify or rule out any venereal diseases and AIDS. I've tried and you can't talk your way out of this one. I had pregnancies less than a year apart and still needed to undergo the entire barrage of screening and testing each and every time. I swear I only had sex with my husband in the past few months, and very infrequently at that, but no dice. A full OB exam is on the agenda. You also have to donate several vials of blood for a full panel and screening to not only measure you health but to assess hormone and viability levels. Most doctors will NOT take this appointment until 8 weeks as the chances of miscarriage before this point is extremely high. This is an

exciting visit. You see and hear your baby. If your husband / partner / significant other / mother / best friend isn't intimidated by the thought of a full exam bring them along. Tell them to shield their eyes or be like a ninja, not heard and not seen during the swabbing, etc. but if they want to concentrate on the ultrasound screen they get a first peek and usually a picture as a souvenir to take home. Very excite, very excite.

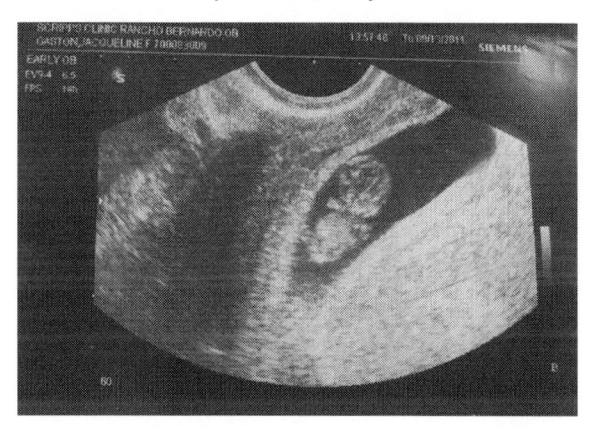

First ultrasound of Jacob

My total exam all 3 times was in several parts:
1) The initial discussion about being pregnant, what type of test you took and when, if you are experiencing any physical issues or problems, and finally when was your last period – OK WRITE THAT DOWN – you are going to have to tell everyone you encounter for the next 9 months when you last period was. So even if you are guessing, guess and write that date down and tell everyone the same date. It's the basis for your preliminary due date calculation. Do yourself a favor and take some time and settle down with a calendar and figure it out. If you were like me, you had been actively trying to get pregnant and know the date off the top of your head.
2) Then disrobe and put on the little paper draping open in the front. It's time for the gynecological exam with swabs and scrapings, etc. Butt at the end of the table, feet in the stirrups, let your legs fall open. Hey isn't that how we got here in the first place?
3) Then the lights went off for the ultrasound. Gloves on and lots of lubricant on a giant dildo shaped probe that's going into your

womanly cavity. Up on the screen you will see your little guy and hear the heartbeat. Takes about 5 minutes but feels like forever. I cried. Each time. When I heard that little heartbeat. That's the moment where if your husband / partner is in the room you just lose it. Your little gift of love has taken root. It's pure joy. It's love. It's elation. Take it in and cry your eyes out.

4) Then clothes back on, and to the nurses station for a quick discussion and your little alien photo as a souvenir to take home. You will get a bag of stuff. Most of it advertising for various baby sites, registries and the start of the endless stream of products you must have. Also a few samples of prenatal vitamins, and list upon lists of things you cannot take like medicines, foods, etc. Finally I got a set of orders to take down to the laboratory.

5) Blood draws at the lab. I vaguely remember giving 4-6 vials that first time. Plus be ready to start giving urine samples at every office visit.

That is about an hour, hour and half from start to finish and it's an emotionally up and down visit and you definitely need a snack and a nap afterwards. I advise bringing some water or maybe even a Gatorade for that. If you are already not feeling so hot giving that much blood may leave you dizzy and a little light headed. It's time to start prepping your pregnancy / parenting purse anyway. Have a granola bar or apple or some kind of snack with you. You may need it badly. I found that things come on so quickly while you are pregnant. Having to go to the bathroom hits like a tidal wave as does nausea and of course the need for sleep and sex.

Tests run: Pregnancy Test (Duh) STD and VD screening, AIDS, blood levels, hormone levels.

Monthly appointments. Depending on your situation the second month's appointments bring the following tests; First Trimester screening and the MaterniT21. The generic typical visit goes as follows;

Weigh in. Depending on the week you are weighed which is so not fun, especially as you are getting bigger. I used to turn the other way on the scale. I had no desire to see my enormous size being legitimized with an actual number on the scale.

Then give a urine sample. This was no problem for me as I had to go to the bathroom every few minutes anyway. I drank some water in the car ride over to prepare then prayed I didn't have to go before I got called back for the appointment. If you do don't sit in the waiting room in distress, tell someone you have to go and a nurse will make sure you get a sample cup.
Go into an exam room and get naked from the waist down. Blood pressure. Very important. Part of this is genetics. I had perfect spot on pressures with all of my pregnancies regardless of weight gain. I'm lucky. Not everyone is. My husband's cousin had a later in life baby and ended up delivering early due to gestational diabetes and blood pressure issues.
Doppler on your belly to hear the heartbeat. Your belly is also measured with a tape measure to make sure you are on track. I aced that one.
Any questions or complaints.

At the end of the appointments I'd met the nurse at her station to go over the next steps. Quite often I would get sent down to the lab for blood work and additional testing such as your trimester screening or glucose test are discussed and scheduled. Sometimes I'd have to arrange to come back another time like to take the test, especially any which require fasting like the glucose test. Others we'd have to schedule at the perinatology department of the hospital such as critical ultrasounds or an amniocentesis. Now OB nurses are insurance savvy and know what requires pre-authorization. The overall intensity of these visits will vary all based on you, your health and the baby. There are appointments leading up to but especially after critical testing and development stages that require more time. This is your routine every month for the next 6 months.

16-18 weeks. Anatomical ultrasound and Amniocentesis. 16-18 weeks.

I had this go 3 different ways during 3 different pregnancies.

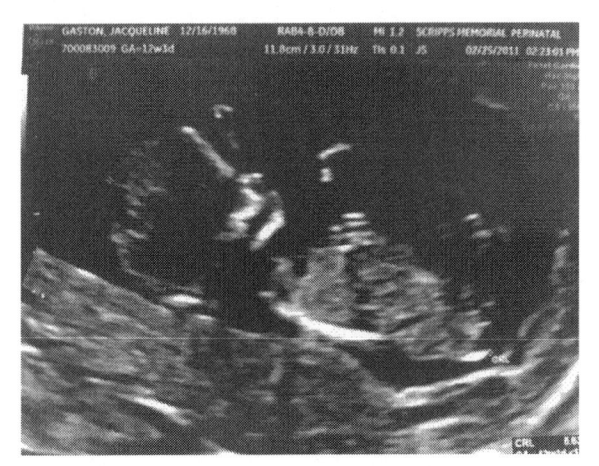

At 18 weeks it's magical it's a baby instead of an alien

Pregnancy 1. Our first amnio appointment was an all day affair at UCSD Medical Center. First we had to go for genetic counseling. We had to wait in a lobby area with about 6 other high risk couples. I was 42 at the time. Some people were older. Some were younger. All couples though. The older couples were dressed very professionally. There was a younger couple and the husband was in a military uniform. There must be something really bad in their genetics or their backgrounds. The questionnaire you fill out asks you to identify any abnormality in any of your direct and indirect relatives. Its pages of grids, does your mother, maternal grandmother, maternal grandfather, father, paternal grandmother, paternal grandfather, brother, sister, cousin, aunt, uncle have diabetes? Cancer? Anyone with a mental illness. It's endless. After waiting for about ½ hour, which is almost how long it took to fill out the paperwork, we went into a back office for genetic counseling. We were taken back into a very bland room were we sat down. I don't know if the person we met with was a doctor but what she did have was a laminated 2 sided sheet with all of the risk factors for all types of genetic disorders and your statistical probabilities as indicated by your age at conception. She spent the next 45 minutes reading us the statistical probability of our baby having every single genetic abnormality they had records of. Are you kidding me? The genetic counseling was one of the worst 45 minutes of my life and left me absolutely terrified as to the outcome of this pregnancy. My husband wanted to punch the counselor as I'm crying on the way out. At my age we have zero change of having a healthy baby. I had always prescribed to the philosophy that a baby, any baby, every baby, was a blessing. I know there are exceptions but all throughout this pregnancy I was so elated to be pregnant, to be having a baby with my husband, and this was a rocket launcher aimed straight at the heart of my balloon of happiness. I've never left an appointment being so depressed and hopeless. I felt like an absolute loser for having gotten pregnant. I knew that having a baby this late in life I was going to be faced with some very difficult decisions if something was wrong. After that meeting it seemed that something being wrong and going wrong was inevitable she didn't even hint at the potential problems that I was going to face. The next doctor did that for me.

After genetic counseling we went into the procedure room and I had an ultrasound. Please keep in mind for these ultrasounds they want your bladder FULL. So I hadn't gone to the bathroom for a few hours after consuming a bunch of water to prep for the test. Agony. Pain. And I hadn't had the big needle yet that I had been dreading. There were 2 necessities in this pregnancy I had been dreading from a fear of needles stand point: the amnio and the inevitable epidural. The thought of these giant needles going into my body scared me more than anything else. First an ultrasound to pinpoint the babies exact location so they don't stab it with the giant needle that will be used to extract your amniotic fluid. I'm laying on the table and the ultrasound is pretty straight forward. Before the actual procedure 2 things happened. The doctor performing the amnio explained the loss risks, that by having this procedure I was putting the baby at risk and there was if I recall correctly a 1 in 400 chance of losing the pregnancy by doing this (or the Mayo clinic sights 0.6% chance.) The other thing I did was sign off on a study that the University I had the test done at was conducting, allowing my blood and some of my embryonic flood to be sampled for a clinical trail developing an assay to try and reduce the need for amnios in the future. Gladly. No brainer. Thank goodness. Very few women in the future will ever have to do what I did, twice I might add. The MaterniT21 assay from Sequenom gives you a full genetic profile from a blood draw from you around week 10. The new test is a game changer. Then here comes the needle. I couldn't look and neither could my husband. You get a swab with the orange antiseptic stuff then a large and I mean 8-10 inch needle is inserted into your belly. There was a sharp pain when the needle went in. It did last a while and felt achy afterwards. Boom. It draws fluid for about 30 seconds then you are done. Looking back it was not the most unpleasant thing that my body went through though at the time it was definitely the scariest. It does hurt but it's not overwhelming. When weighing this discomfort, which intensely physically lasts a minute then residual aches for a few hours, against having a definitive genetic profile and have a huge degree of certainty that things are ok, over 99% it's worth it every single time. It's not like toothache hurt or, as you will find, the beginning of labor pains hurt. I remember the most discomfort feeling the fluid being drawn. When the needle comes out and you get a band aid, no lollypop though, bitches, and sit for a minute, get dressed and the results will be ready in 4-10 days. The recovery for the amnio is not terrible. Don't strain yourself and take it easy for a day or two

Waiting a week for the results was even worse especially after the genetic counseling. An amnio is one of those procedures that makes you want to lay in bed for the rest of the day. During my first 2 pregnancies I battled not only physical but mental exhaustion. The stress and strain of dealing with a one in two chance of having a baby with a serious issue, and having to have an amnio draw which in itself runs a risk of terminating your pregnancy through complication, and then having to wait for the results and having only a few days to make a decision if you want to go forward with your pregnancy or not based on the results, its mind blowing how crazy insane that is. That time I had a week. A week, once the results were going to come in to terminate the pregnancy if there was a problem, within the law. 20 weeks is the cut off for a 'termination' and even then the doctors won't do it you have to go to Planned Parenthood to get that done. A week to contact other experts try to get a second opinion and to decide if you are going to end this pregnancy and move on or keep going. I have friends who faced with all of the screening and counseling decided to leave things in God's hands. I have another friend who when you tell her this she says nonsense. God created the doctors who created the procedures that allow you to know what is going on and be prepared. I received a phone call the next week letting me know everything looked good and no genetic abnormalities were detected. Phew.

Pregnancy 2: I couldn't have been more high risk going into this pregnancy. I was old and just had a loss. Went to a different facility this time. Scripps Hospital in La Jolla who has a pretty extensive perinatal department with high resolutions ultrasound and a perinatalogist on call daily. Waved off the genetic counseling. All of the statistics from the previous visit were already burned in my head and with everyday as I was getting older I was also moving closer and closer to having a baby with real problems. So I went straight in for the ultrasound. I had been bleeding a little that month, spotting, turned out I had a uterine tear and it was decided at that time I should wait 1-2 weeks before trying to do the procedure. As previously discussed the risk of loss due to the amnio its self is decent, but with this uterine tear the fear was I would lose too much fluid or start bleeding excessively. So time was to be given for the tear to heal. The problem with that was that I was potentially going to get the results right before the legal time limit to terminate the pregnancy. I wasn't going to have a whole lot of options if I decided that the issues with the baby were so overwhelming that I didn't want to go forward. In the meantime I had the full anatomical ultrasound which takes about an hour. Again you have to have a full bladder and it's kind of agonizing to have the ultrasound probe pressed against your belly to get good readings when your bladder is painfully full. The facility I went to had a bathroom in the ultrasound room so as soon as they have the pictures and readings that meet the requirements you can relieve yourself. They look at the fingers and toes. They measure the baby's femur. They look exhaustively at the skull and spine. The heartbeat is tracked. Takes 30-45 minutes to get all of the images they need to look at.

I went back almost 2 weeks later and the tear had healed to the point where the doctor felt good about performing the amnio. This is where having certain medical team members you really trust comes into play. This doctor, who was all of 4'9" in heels, where as I am almost 6 feet tall in flip flops, was my perinatal rock. I trusted her, I had faith in her decisions and guidance. This is critical when you are talking about a procedure that person is going to do, their hands with a needle in them penetrating your uterus to collect a sample, and that you might lose your baby because of this, you need someone you have total faith in that doctor. We were quite a pair walking down the halls together going to discuss test results, with the foot plus height discrepancy, but she became my friend, my advocate, and a champion for me not having an amnio on my last pregnancy. She also helped expedite my amnio results since we were so close to the 20 week mark. She called me a few days later with the initial results, this was the ONE time that a call from the doctor with test results was a good thing not a bad one. I then got the remaining results a few days after that. Relief.

Pregnancy 3: Because I had the MaterniT21 test I did not have to have an amnio. That was determined after the perinatalogist read the results from my prior testing and saw all of the views on the anatomical ultrasound. I had a wiggly kid who moved the whole time until they needed to get a ton of views of her spine and she got into a position that the technician couldn't coax her out of despite all of the tricks so I had to come back to complete the pictures the following week. Coming back down to the hospital for a second anatomical ultrasound, 1000% better than having an amnio.

During that first real anatomical ultrasound you usually get a decent set of photos. Some people frame them. It's one of the largest and most important landmarks in your pregnancy. Test results are one thing, but seeing the baby's heart beat and watching him or her move, that is something else. It's not an unpleasant procedure except that your bladder is really full and that can cause some sharp pains while the probe is being pressed and moved around on your belly.

30-32 weeks. Final ultrasound. Everything good? I had one good one and one not so good one. During both of my last ultrasounds the good news was the baby looked great. The babies were both in ready to deliver position. Head down ready to go. Always a relief. I've heard that when you have to have intervention to get a baby out of breach to avoid a c-section it's absolute agony. Now my yoga instructor swore by a holistic approach involving stretches and maneuvers to help the baby rotate. She also touted a routine that allowed women to have a vaginal birth after caesarian. I would have signed up for all of that if I had those issues. I would try anything to avoid surgery. Anything.

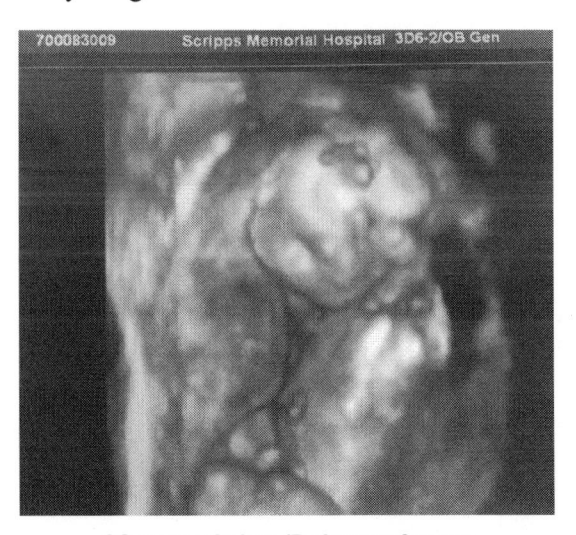

SO creepy, the best 4D ultrasound we got

Ultrasounds in general. I've had my share. The clinic where my doctor is has a few options. One in the ob/gyn department that is ok resolution. Another higher end down in the basement. They also have a policy that the ultrasound technician cannot interpret any results or discuss any findings. So you are in room with a person during a pretty intimate moment and they can't tell you anything. They can give you instruction so they can get all of the views they need but cannot make any other comment. I've had ultrasounds at 2 different hospitals in the perinatology departments on the super high end resolution variety. It's up on a big screen for you to see. A giant 60" TV. Those technicians do discuss observations with you and I found them to be extremely pleasant and personable.

I must confess I held my breath during every ultrasound I had until I saw or heard the baby's heartbeat. There were some terrifying moments. Occasionally the technicians have to root around to find the baby and get the heartbeat up. Some of them I didn't even look at the screen at all during the procedure. Having a loss takes the potential enjoyment out of seeing your baby in the womb. With my son I had monthly ultrasounds. I was able to cut that down with my last pregnancy after getting 'medical street credit' for having successfully carried and delivered my son with no issues.

Who to take? You can't take kids to an ultrasound. You can't take kids to a pelvic exam. My husband is a love and came with me to 85% of my appointments. The ones he didn't come to weren't ultra critical. I made sure he was there at 8 weeks, the anatomical ultrasound and the 3rd trimester ultrasound. The appointments towards the end of your pregnancy he was there for most of them. My mom offered to come but instead I had her babysit while I went alone if my husband was unavailable. I did have 1 appointment that I regretted not having him at. It was a perinatal ultrasound during the middle of my 2nd pregnancy, which was considered the most high risk since I had had a loss at 6 months into my first pregnancy. I had to drive myself about 45 minutes to the hospital. Wait and have the ultrasound, meet with the perinatalogist and drive myself home. I was physically and emotionally exhausted and that drive home was absolutely miserable. Now I'm a tough girl. A Viking as it were. I felt very weak and vulnerable. One of the few times in my life my insides were saying "please take pity on me" because I was so old and pregnant and tired and beat.

36-40 weeks. Weekly appointments. Escalated monthly exams. Weight. Urine. Blood pressure. Then mine consisted of fetal monitoring for about 30 minutes looking for activity. You sit in a pleather recliner with a monitor on your belly and a jeopardy signaling device in your hand. When you feel a kick you hit the button. Here is what they are looking for: the babies heartbeat recovery after activity. Apparently this is an indicator if the baby is having any trouble or issues at this stage. If you don't have a lot of movement the nurse will hit you with a cattle prod type device in the belly until the baby moves. Not kidding. It actually is a big buzzer that must scare the Jesus out of the little one. Not a peaceful or tranquil test though it gives the illusion of being because it's boring as hell and you are sitting in a makeshift recliner and your husband or mine I should say was on his phone checking ESPN scores while you sit in this room behind a shower curtain for ½ hour or longer. Then a quick dilation check. It's the beginning of everyone sticking fingers in your vagina. It doesn't stop until you've had the baby or very shortly there after. Do NOT panic if you aren't dilated at your doctor's appointments. Labor really does vary for everyone and someone may be decently dilated for a few weeks, 2 to 3cm and start labor late or having a ridiculously long labor. It doesn't indicate much except that your body is starting to get ready. I thought it was one of those things where the doctor is like 'as long as you are here and naked lets check under the hood.' Ehhh. Also a Doppler sound on the heartbeat. That's always nice and comforting. Finally a quick low resolution ultrasound where basic and very rough measurements are taken calculate the amniotic fluid volumes. They are looking for too little. Sometimes fluid does leak and sometimes there is a problem. Low fluid is a very big deal and if the levels are too low expect you will be taken to the hospital immediately for monitoring and possibly an emergency c-section. Along with the heartbeat recovery of the baby is the most important parts of the visit. With my final high risk pregnancy this went up to twice a week. Total drag but I guess better safe than sorry. I actually was painfully resentful that nothing more than my age made my life stop for those last weeks and I was a slave to coming in for testing. Age discrimination, not cool.

8. Testing and Screenings.
Are We Having Fun Yet ?!?

Things have changed even in the short time since my first pregnancy to writing this book. With my first pregnancy I underwent a battery of tests, mostly specific to the trimester I was in. First trimester is the blood work for any STD's, AIDs, etc. Over the course of your pregnancy you will give endless vials of blood. You will lose any fear of giving blood and needles pretty quickly. You are given an gynecological exam during your initial pregnancy visit along with an internal ultrasound. This is to get baselines and to make sure you are healthy and disease free going in. Finally your hormone levels are assessed to make sure your body is producing enough progesterone etc. to sustain your pregnancy properly. Since I was I don't know the consequence of not being so.

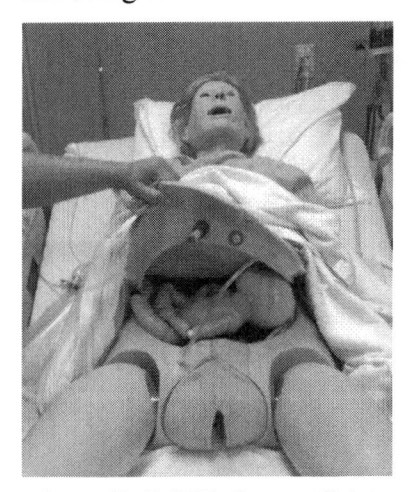

Source: Noelle ™ The Pregnant Robot

A very flawed screening that hopefully will go by the way of the dinosaurs is the first trimester screening. Not only is it not covered by insurance, it's a mandatory California screening to I believe identify your risk of Down's Syndrome and the baby having an extra set of chromosomes. It is sent out to a state run lab, hence why your insurance won't cover it and it's a complete pain in the ass to deal with the billing and payments. Anyway the test is flawed in that your age is a factor. Every screening I took came back positive and as it was explained to me that just means that there is a risk and additional testing is warranted. Several months later your bill shows up. It states that you don't have insurance and if you'd like to submit the bill for insurance fill out the back and send it back in. Ok. Then a few more months later you get a statement saying your insurance won't cover it. Which they usually don't, it's a straight up 3rd party lab that isn't in network. Twice I wasn't able to resolve the billing until after I delivered. Once I had the pleasure of waiting on hold for an hour to try and speak with someone who could only tell me that processing took 8-12 weeks and couldn't tell me any specifics of my billing status. The only reason I actually called is because I kept getting past due notices in the mail regarding this bill but if they accepted my insurance or not was still 'pending'. I know I overpaid once. By $40 or something like that. I never received any refund. **Update. Almost 2 years later I received a call from a nice lady from the state of California. She said I am owed a credit of about $150. I said I know exactly what this is for. She said you wouldn't believe how many people have no clue. I explained that I received the bill and paid it because it said it was overdue already (that is one of the fun parts of all of the medical billing is by the time the bill is processed and sent it's already over due or due immediately.) So I sent a payment before my insurance was processed. Two years later. More than two years. Do you believe that? I am going to spend my money on something nice for the kids. The bad news the very nice lady told me was that is was going to take 8-12 weeks for my check to arrive. Something is better than nothing. I'll spend it all at Target in 10 minutes.

In addition to the blood work, which is extensive, add in ultrasounds. Fetal heart monitoring. The nasty glucose test. Thank goodness the lab I went to chilled it. You go in. Drink a nasty flat orange soda tasting drink. Have a blood draw an hour later. If you pass great. If you don't it's another round. The butt swipe at the end of your pregnancy to test for strep B. This fun filled test is executed by taking a swab of your butt for processing. I actually didn't know I tested positive until I was in the hospital in labor with my son. I had to have a bag of IV antibiotics on board immediately to reduce the risk of transfer to my little one. Ewww and ewww. My contaminated ass had to be dealt with. While delivering my daughter I had the same issue, I had tested positive again. However she came out so fast and furious there was NO time to get a bag of antibiotics on board. Another battery of testing was then required to clear her including blood tests, seeing the on call pediatrician at the hospital twice who had to clear her before she was released and bringing her in to see my pediatrician on day 3 for further evaluation and follow up.

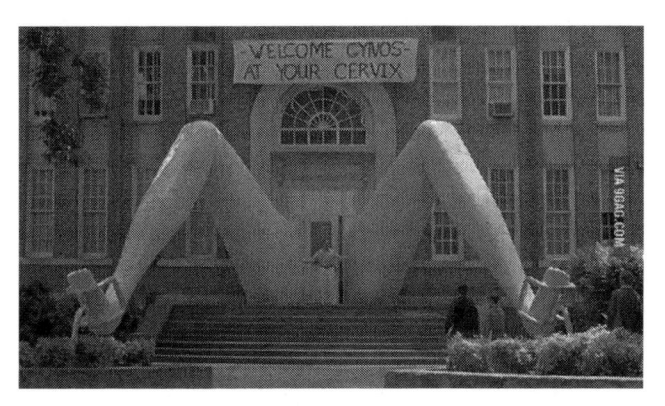

Movie "Patch Adams:" Universal Studios 1999

Heads up on testing. Again if a nurse calls you, everything is great no problems, passed with flying colors. One of the hardest waiting periods of my life was waiting for my MaterniT21test for my 3rd pregnancy. When my doctor's nurse called not a week later the sigh of relief was so extreme. I was in the clear. I could eliminate 7 months of worry. No genetic issues. Thank you Jesus. Our nurse then asked to speak with my husband during the results phone call and told him the gender, since I was trying not to find out. I had a healthy boy at that point and a daughter via marriage so I wanted to be surprised. Not finding out actually lasted about 2 weeks before I overheard my husband talking to a friend and the cat was out of the bag. No the concern is when it's the doctor calling. They usually have really packed schedules so when they take the time to call you keep in mind it's usually because the situation is bigger than the nurse handles from a liability stand point. It's usually not great news, not horrible, but usually a bad result on test or screening. If you see your doctor's office calling, pick it up, right away. Once you let it go to voicemail and the doctor has to leave a message, during which you aren't going to get specific information, just a request to call him back, their schedules really are crazy with patients and hospital rounds that it's very difficult to get a hold of them again. Which just fuels your anxiety. I've had two of those doctor calls. They are no fun.

With the test and the screenings and the unending ob and prenatal appointments there still is this vast vacuum of time that for me was filled with never ending anxiety. Fear and stress over what I was eating, what I had eaten and how that would effect my baby's brain development now and in the future. About all of the times I had partied, smoked, drank, and how that was going to effect my baby today and tomorrow. The articles about eating this and not eating that. Oh my gosh I had a hot dog, now what. I ate some lunchmeat and didn't microwave it first. Listeria for sure. You have to realize that the doctor's even know that you are going to eat things that are on the do not eat list and do things that are on the do not do list. No one follows the instructions to the letter and there is wiggle room. Having said that I feel like I did my best to adhere to all of the rules and I took it seriously and yes I did cheat now and then and I probably could have done a better job keeping my weight down and my fitness up but hell it was a party, a celebration, and I let myself indulge.

Glucose Test: To screen for gestational diabetes and make sure you body is still regulating your sugar correctly. Administered around your 6th month. Separate from your monthly exam you schedule an appointment with the lab. You go in on an empty stomach so try to get an appointment first thing in the morning. First a blood draw as a base sugar level. Then you drink a small bottle of viscous liquid that tastes like flat Sunkist soda. Our lab is benevolent and chills theirs so it's palatable. Then you wait an hour and have another blood draw. Done.

I did not follow a diet while pregnant. I stayed off the do not eat list for fear of hurting the baby, well for the most part, but I indulged and mostly in sweets. I did not see a blip in my glucose level during any pregnancies. I ate everything, donuts, cake, ice cream, shamrock shakes, you name it I ate it. Little Debbie's

Swiss Cake Rolls, best served chilled. Could eat a whole box. Yum. Didn't blip my glucose. My husband's cousin is my age and we were pregnant together during my first pregnancy. She developed gestational diabetes and ended up delivering 3 weeks early because of it. As with many pregnancy complications and symptomology, part of it is genetics. What the doctors are trying to mitigate are the controllable factors, which are VERY slim and finite. Don't do crack. Don't drink , well not too much they say now. Things that have proven in the past to have a sliver of negative side effects to your developing off spring. Otherwise it's a crap shoot based on YOU and you alone, not your mamma, not your aunt, not your mother in law, YOU and your genetics and dispositions. I've seen so many different women have such vastly different pregnancies. A friend of my husbands once told me while she was pregnant with her 3rd in 4 years that her body wasn't made for carrying babies. That every time she had such bad side effects she required IV's and hospitalization just for her to stay healthy even in the first trimester. She was out on disability for most of her pregnancies. Conversely I've known women who don't even have a ripple in their existence while pregnant and work up until their due dates. A lot of that depends on your constitution. I was fine during my first pregnancies but opted to take it easy because I was such high risk. I slept a lot. Took it easy in general. My last pregnancy was physically my hardest. I was sick, I was exhausted, I kept getting sick, I hurt all over, I had insane volcanic acid reflux, I was a mess. If you don't know what round ligament pain is call me. If you don't know that all of those hormones meant to help your ligaments 'relax' so you deliver can wreak havoc with your joints, call me. I was a gassy bloated puky fever having acid reflux in total continuous pain monster with my last, but I forged on as I had a toddler to run after. I've seen women on the strictest of diets gain an ungodly amount of weight and have all kinds of health issues. I've seen gluttonous women like myself eat everything not have an issues and after my son I lost all of the weight within 6 months. Not bad without the benefit of having a celebrity trainer.

Genetic Counseling. Here is a small part of the limitless facts that are presented to you during your first genetic counseling session.

Maternal Age at Delivery and Risk of Down Syndrome or Similar Chromosomal Birth Defect	
Maternal Age (Years)	**Chromosomal Birth Defect** *
>25-29	>2
>30-34	>3
>35	>5
>36	>6
>37	>8
>38	>10
>40	>16
>41	>20
>45	>50
Source: Center for Disease Control Division of Birth Defects and Developmental Disabilities, NCBDDD, Centers for Disease Control and Prevention	

Is that enough to scare you yet? Maybe into getting a dog instead of having a baby? I don't blame you. This is where the pavement meets the road. What that says is that after 45 you have a 1 in 2 chance of having a baby with Down's Syndrome. I was 42 at the time of my one and only session. It was horrifying. Followed by an amnio. Double fun double header day. My sister is a PhD and I called her afterwards crying. She assured me that the statistics are just numbers and do not apply to the individual. By having had 2 perfectly healthy children over the age of 43 I have done by part to improve those statistics even if only by a fraction. They are daunting, haunting, and before the MaterniT21 test which is now available at week 10 of your pregnancy, waiting the 18 weeks for an amnio then another 2 for the results is harrowing. Once those results come in you have less than a week to terminate your pregnancy if that is your choice. The fact that these are deadlines you need to consider adds just another level of stress to an already stressful high risk pregnancy.

All of the testing, imaging, blood draws, doctor's appointments, and racking up fees and medical bills I'm happy to say fade into the distance after your baby comes. Some bills from your pregnancy care will linger, but you won't care as much. All of the testing is to track the health of you and your baby so try to relax and do you best to process it all without stressing out too much. It is hard, but you can do it because the outcome is totally worth it.

9. Weight Gain. Reaching Goodyear Blimp Status.

The other day I was out and about and ran into a very pregnant lady. She was telling me how her doctor was warning her that she was gaining too much weight and needed to be careful. At 8 months she had gained a little less than 30 pounds. What? Even her husband was pissed at that advice. Now I didn't go into the specifics so I can't say for sure but she was really dumbfounded and confused when I told her I had gained about 70 each time as did many of my friends. I've found that weight gain goes in 2 categories. The fit and lean who are going to stay fit and lean and maybe a few babies in are going to get really big in that last month to the point where they look almost unnatural but for the most part are staying under the 30 pound mark and don't look pregnant from behind and are going to bounce back pretty quick. Most of these women are pretty slight as well. Short and small in stature. The woman in question was at her pre-baby weight and body less than 3 months after delivery. She's very petite and lean. Being a bigger person to begin with, almost 6 feet tall with an optimal weight being over 150, I guess I didn't see weight gain the same way. If I started at 170 and gained 70 I guess it's similar to starting at 115 and gaining around 30. It took a while also before people could tell I was pregnant and not just gaining weight. Over the summer my neighbor was on her second in three years, she stayed really slight for quite a while. She did get a little basketball belly in month 3 but not very big until month 8 then her belly was almost as big as the rest of her proportionally speaking. I gauge weight loss based on the following: how old you are, how much you weighed before hand and what your goal is. My goal was to be happy, healthy and have a perfect baby. My mission was more than accomplished.

With all of my weight gain my blood pressure didn't blip and my glucose levels weren't effected. Another "scientific" study was released saying that if you gain too much weight while pregnant and spike your glucose levels are you seriously increasing the risk of having an obese child. That you should only gain 40 pounds or less. Get the heck out of here with that. For real. Kids today are obese because they eat a bunch of garbage and don't exercise.

They spend too much time on their phones and playing video games and not just going outside and working up a sweat. They are just like me while pregnant except I'm an adult and I know that I need to steer the boat in the other direction after the baby comes. I can't imagine the harm these scientific studies are going to end up doing. Coupled with celebrities having babies and looking like a million bucks a week later my money is on there being a string of undernourished babies or women who develop bulimia while pregnant, which will be classified as a new syndrome and in need of a slew of scientific studies, and more harm than good will come out of this new weight restriction. In China decades ago the society decided boys were the most desirable child to have. The government then put a restriction of one child per family. Without going into too much minutia, women are the most desired commodity in China to the point where the really refined and sophisticated women want NOTHING to do with Chinese men because they are spoiled babies. Stupid restrictions backfire. An important lesson for all parents to learn. The more you make something forbidden and give it meaning by being bad the more your kids will be attracted to it. On a smaller level I have outlet covers all over our house. What this has done with our second baby is actually attract her to the outlets and she quickly figured out how to take the covers out, stick them in her mouth, and try to stick them back in. So what's worse? No cover or a potentially preventative measure that ends up backfiring. Applies to a lot of scenarios. Except eating well, exercising, brushing your teeth and learning manners. In all 4 of those areas all work is good work and nothing bad comes from brushing your teeth and exercising. Well maybe but seriously it's rare and you have to be a little OCD to take those tenants to a bad place.

I also just saw a newsletter from my prenatal yoga instructor. She, as I would imagine your yoga instructor as well, is an amazing resource during your pregnancy. The newsletter was about helping with post partum depression. I've always felt that a lot of issues, and especially disappointments regarding the entire spectrum of experience of having a baby can eased by managing expectations and skewing your mindset. One way is with your weight. Am I happy that I'm still 20-30 pounds heavier than my ideal weight almost a year and half after my last baby? Not really but I'm also not terribly sad about it either. I knew I was going to gain weight. I knew I wanted to eat what I wanted to eat. I know that having a house full of kids means having cabinets full of kid food. I know that I don't spend enough time working out and that I could push harder. But I'm ok with all of it. I didn't mind gaining weight while pregnant at all. In fact it was kind of cool. There is nothing more womanly to me than having big full boobs and a belly and a crazy juicy butt. It's the thigh and bat flap arms I could live without but the rest of it, love love love.

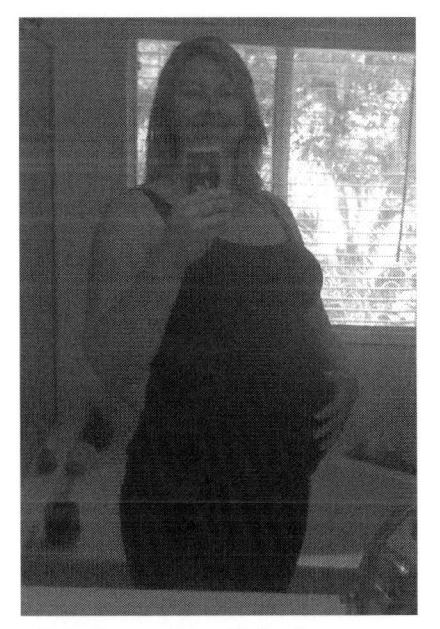

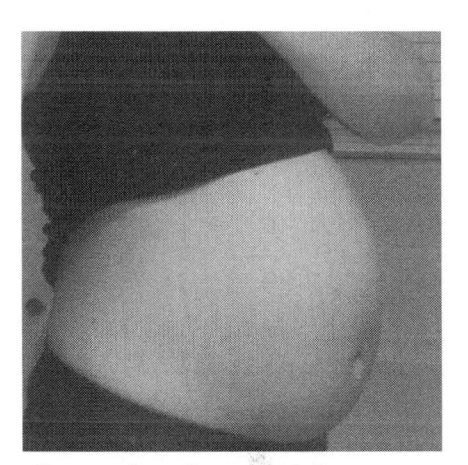

Gorgeous 8 month pregnant belly

8 months pregnant with Jacob

I also realized though it's a bit of a tough pill to swallow now that being older and eating whatever I wanted and not really exercising hard and getting pregnant and having babies was going to leave me a bit fat and out of shape. Oh well. My litmus test is does my husband still want to do me? If the answer is yes than we are good to go. I don't need to break out my pre-pregnancy bikini's for a photo shoot. That's where I think most women have the disconnect. Their expectations are not realistic based on the celebrity examples that are prolific in the media. A recent high profile mom to be was Coco Austin, Ice-T's wife. She spent her pregnancy denying rumors that she was using a surrogate because she gained less than 20 pounds total and walked out of the hospital basically looking like herself already. Even Princess Kate walked out of the hospital with a baby belly and she is a thin ass woman. A recent quote from Anne Hathaway challenged this fad of celebrity moms looking amazing 4 weeks later saying that your body isn't supposed to go back the way it was. That everything has changed as it should since you just created another human being. Preach girl. Now someone like Coco is super curvy and it goes back to my point about how your body was before. If you are slight, small in stature you are going to feel every pound. Being a larger as Eric Cartman would describe "big boned" woman I don't feel anything until I gain at least 10 pounds and even then it's not significant. I feel 10 pounds now, after babies, on my knees and joints as I'm exercising but not so much in my clothes.

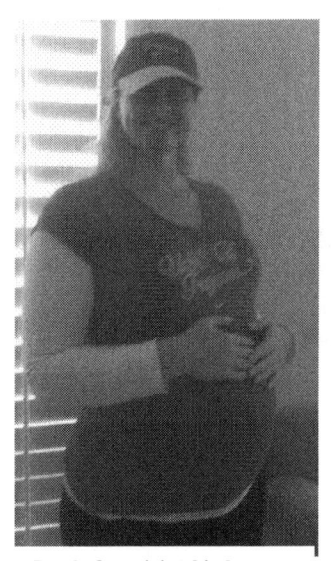

Day before giving birth

Along those lines everyone is different. Some women see their pregnancy as a point of joy, some as a job, some as a license to eat, put me in that category, oh and the joy one too, and others as a minor inconvenience. Those are the ones that see their kids that way too btw. But as previously stated I'm always surprised by how stupefied and confused most women seem when I talk to them about specific issues. I guess I could consider myself to have an above average confidence level but some of the basics seem just that, basic and that everyone should know about them. I can also say that if a doctor told me that 30 pounds was too much to gain while pregnant my first reaction would be well what do they know? If I don't have any other adverse effects of the weight gain who cares but me and my husband. How do women not know these things? Doctor's aren't gods, just like me being a confident person doesn't make me an expert at anything other than my own personal experience. I can give you a list of things I think are important but they are important to me and me alone. I hope it helps and gives you some insight but my expertise is solely based on my experiences.

I can't tell you how many things can go wrong or sideways but maintaining your expectations I felt was the key to happiness. I had no focus what so ever on the means of delivery. I wanted to have an epidural, got one with my first. I didn't want to have a c-section, managed that. But seriously as long as the baby was healthy I didn't care if someone took me by my feet and turned me upside down and shook me until my baby came out. I was not married to the means, just the outcome. Same with my post pregnancy body and child care. At some point you are going to be an adult and a parent and you are going to have to trust yourself. You are going to trust your judgment and your decisions. Getting in tune with your body isn't a bad plan either. I see so many women who are so upset and hating on themselves after pregnancy for that extra 15 pounds they can't get rid of, or the notion that they no longer can wear a bikini. Boo hoo. Seriously. Is your baby healthy and thriving, then can it. White Girl Problems 101. "Pumpkin Spice Latte for Crystal in the Uggh boots." As you move forward in your journey there are going to be tens if not hundreds of teachers, doctors, family members, even strangers who want to give you their two cents about what you should be doing and how to raise your children. Now might be a good time to grow a backbone and learn to not only be an advocate for yourself but for your child. If you can present a positive confident front your child will look up to you as an expert. Children want a strong parental figure. Not a friend, not someone who is wishy-washy and insecure but a momma tiger fighting for her young. Be that.

Embrace that. I'm confounded by women who are scared and unsure. This is NOT the time for that. I'm taken aback by women who don't want to gain too much weight because their husbands don't like them fat. Ladies, screw that clown, it's not about him its about you. If you are going to be hating on yourself for stretch marks, or hips that won't go back down in place how are you supposed to be happy and enjoy the beautiful gift of parenthood. Your body isn't supposed to be the same after babies. You just created life and there are side effects. There was a fat substitute called Olestra and the commercials used to talk about anal leakage. It's a lot like that. So your slim fit American Eagle low riders jeans are out. Embrace the high waited compression Capri black yoga pant. So you've got more hips and butt now for your husband to paw it. If gaining weight and having mustard gas caliber farts that make your husband choke and you are afraid of pooping while giving birth, then maybe fostering or adopting is for you. I have to tell you if you think that's bad wait until you have that baby. You will be on bio-hazard clean up duty for a long, long time and even today I'm surprised and borderline sickened by some of the monstrosities that come out of my children's sphincters. If you believe the hype pregnancy symptoms are just a prep for the main even to come. Again as Eric Cartman would say, the appetizer is what you eat before you eat to make you more hungry.

10. Our Loss. Baby Grace.

Ok so the first time I got pregnant I'm not sure I did anything right. First off I got pregnant on my birthday weekend. My birthday where I turned 42, well past my baby having prime if you believe what you read. My future husband and I were partying hard with our friends. I was smoking and drinking. I believe we stayed up for 36 hours straight. I vaguely remember my husband practically passed out in the hot tub as the sun was coming up. While I had been prepping to get pregnant, neither my eating nor my lifestyle habits were totally on point. About 2 weeks later before I knew I was pregnant I had a dental x-ray. I also ended up with a ton of stress in my life. Stress from my husbands ex-wife who threatened to rescind all of his custody when she found I was pregnant, to the stress of my husband's buddy and daughter who stayed with us for the first four months of my pregnancy. He was going through a nasty divorce and he was really out of it and needed help.

Those were the negatives. The pluses were that I was super fit going in, beyond fit. I had support from my work which I was a part owner in along with my parents who were going to have their first blood related grandchild. I had the best medical care you could. We had a high end PPO and I had every test done that first few months that you could, from vials and vials of blood being drawn for screenings to an amnio and ultrasounds. You name it, I had it done. Didn't help though. After waiting that precautionary period of really not telling anyone until after 8 weeks then not telling anyone other than family until after the amnio came back clear I still ended up with a loss. The baby died inside me after the 5th month. What did I do wrong? I sat sobbing uncontrollably in the waiting room for the ultrasound of doom. My doctor's primary nurse comforting me. What did I do wrong? The answer was nothing. You can't help but beat yourself up. Was is that dental x-ray? The partying the weekend I got pregnant, the Swiss Cake rolls? My age? My husband's age? I pray that very few people reading this book have to go through this experience, but I'm going to document it step by step anyway because again unless you've been through it you don't know what's involved.

I found out on a Friday afternoon that the baby was not alive. I had no clue. I thought I even been feeling movement. More than likely it was my body cramping or getting ready to expel this little one. It took about 2 hours to confirm that the baby was indeed dead. At first we went into our appointment and met with the nurse practitioner since our doctor was not in the office that day. This set the tone for the next few years as I would dread meeting with anyone other than MY doctor, it filled me with despair. The nurse practitioner measured my stomach and said it looked a little small and had anyone talked to me about the baby being under sized. No they hadn't. Again I had already cleared all of the critical testing and had ultrasounds and an amnio and was given 2 big thumbs up. Then she did the Doppler and couldn't find the heartbeat. She tried changing out the batteries and even went and got a different Doppler from a different room. I was put in the ultrasound room in the OB section and again no heartbeat nor movement detected. My doctor's nurse, Kathy, took me downstairs to the main ultrasound for the clinic. Crying, hysterical. Oh my god! What did I do wrong? Nothing she said. She was an absolute angel. I had to wait in the lounge area for about 10 minutes to go back. I was with a few people who looked like they were undergoing chemotherapy. I was a complete disaster, with Kathy's arm around my shoulder and handing me tissues. The ultrasound tech was not quite a warm fuzzy peach. She claimed she wasn't allowed to tell me anything, that she was only allowed to take images but they had to be read by a doctor. I'm crying, I'm a disaster. She won't give me even a hint of what was going on. That took about 20 minutes.

Finally the loss was confirmed but another OB and I was scheduled into L&D the next day. I was completely inconsolable and my husband was now in charge of listening and getting all of the information we needed. He was given the number of the labor and delivery unit of the hospital associated with our medical clinic. The physicians assistant who had been working with us had called down there and spoke with one of the doctor's on call. My husband then spoke with that doctor and arranged for us to check into labor and delivery the first thing the next morning. We went home, I was an absolute mess. The lowlight was my husband found me laying on the floor in our bathroom just sobbing. Broken hearted. Dying inside. My husband called my parents and told them what was going on. They were on their way back from a week long vacation. They were destroyed.

I did not sleep. I was crying and devastated all night. My husband did not sleep either. The next morning we got up around 6 am and I took a shower and we drove down to the hospital. It's about a ½ hour drive from our house. I don't remember it. I also don't remember checking in. I remember having a very large private room. I had to take my clothes off and change into a gown. I was placed on a labor and delivery table and an IV was started. I remember this room had a curtain partition where the nurses countertop / work area was. The drill was I was going to have to be induced. The induction involved having a suppository placed in my vagina by one of the nurses. Not fun, didn't hurt but felt weird. And yes, yuck. Because I wasn't going to be having a live birth I was offered quite a few drugs to ease the pain. I was given something pretty strong through my IV. By 10am I was in and out of sleep. I was having my progress checked on a pretty regular basis. I wasn't making much and I believe I had a second pitocin suppository a few hours later. By this time my parents and my sister and brother in law were with me. My husband was stationed in a chair next to my bed. He got up from time to time to get coffee but he stayed his post, diligently. Nurses and doctors were coming in and out. All saying the same thing. After some small talk they all reiterated that they weren't supposed to tell us but we should try again right away. This was my only induction, with my two other babies I went into labor on my own. Being induced sucks. I'd say it's far more painful than your body having natural labor. I foolishly thought that the baby was so small I wouldn't need an epidural. By mid afternoon after being pretty heavily medicated I started making some progress and I woke up from my haze in extreme pain. I talked to the nurse and she suggested an epidural, which I was petrified of. Having a big old needle in my spine was at the time worse to me than anything else, must more menacing than the amnio I had a few months before. But the pain had gotten to the threshold were it cut through all of the heavy narcotics I was getting in the IV. I agreed and the anesthesiologist was in our room within the hour. I was in the middle of a pretty horrific event and all I could focus on was how scared I was of having an epidural. You are asked to lean forward and arch your back. You are asked not to move. Oh my gosh is that scary. What if I have to sneeze. I was so tense and concerned about accidentally moving because now I was in labor. I had my husband grab onto my hands so my legs are in front of me and I'm bent in half arching my back and the anesthesiologist is behind me. First lidocaine is injected into the area. Ouch. That pinches and hurts a bit. Then a large needle is placed, that takes about 15-30 seconds to make sure it's placed property. Then a catheter is threaded into your spine. I can't say that hurt, but it was scary and I was anxious about it and it felt very weird. Then you are hooked up to a machine that regularly injects medication into your spine. Took me about 15 minutes for the pain to completely ease off and for the feeling to completely leave my legs and lower extremities.

I can't remember if it was before or after but you have to have a catheter inserted into your urethra to collect your urine because you lose all of the feeling below your waist. Ok that was no fun either. They use some lubricant and the nurse asks you to open your legs and relax, umm yeah right. A small tube is threaded into an area I didn't think you could do that through. It must have been before the epidural now that I think about it because you have to control your legs. Anyway I'm now in labor, not crazy over the top painful labor but regular contracting labor. I'm still in a drugged out haze, fading in and out for the rest of the day. My family members are sitting vigil in my room and my husband is by my side. My family calls it a night at some point and my husband goes to the cafeteria for a cup of coffee. The day has been an absolute blur. I vaguely remember the parade of nurses and doctors coming in. Everyone somber but encouraging that we are such a lovely couple and we shouldn't let this experience deter us from trying again. The doctor on call would come in an introduce themselves to us on shift change. I could hear some of the other women in the unit screaming in pain during delivery. I could hear babies crying. I start to feel funny and I ask the nurse to go get my husband. As he's arriving I feel a giant sploosh between my legs. It was not painful. I just felt something wet pass through me.

Sploosh. As he's approaching the table the nurse lifts up the sheet that has been covering my lower half to confirm that I have in fact delivered. To this day I don't know what my husband did and didn't see. I've never had the guts to ask him. At best he saw a bloody mass on the table, at worst he saw the outline of the baby. A few more nurses and the doctor came in. I still had to deliver the placenta which came out quickly. The baby was immediately taken out of the room and the on call doctor performed a down and dirty examination / autopsy in the hallway to see if she could easily ascertain what had caused my baby to die. She came back about 10 minutes later and said it was clear that the cord had become knotted and shut off. That unless I wanted a more thorough investigation that she didn't feel it was necessary to have a full autopsy performed. How odd that was such a relief. I also had to meet with a social worker on this same topic. Because I was over 20 weeks the standard policy is that the body is released to the parents for burial. The social worker took pity on me and made a decision based on the baby's weight, which had been low, that we didn't meet that criteria. Another factor in this situation was the baby had been tracking small, due to a two vessel cord which is missing a second artery. I didn't know much about this until the baby had already died. It does increase fetal death by a certain percent but usually isn't a main issue and in this case while the baby was tracking small a knot in the cord is what cause her demise. Yes it was a little girl and we had named her Grace.

After delivery and doctor visit my husband went down to the cafeteria with some vouchers and got me some food. I hadn't been allowed to, nor had I wanted to, eat up until that point. I had the best Caesar salad and fruit parfait I'd ever eaten. I was relieved. I was exhausted. I wasn't sad as much as I was just deflated. It was over. So after the social worker visit which allowed me to sign off on the baby being incinerated instead of discharging her to a funeral home for burial, and the doctor reassured us that this was a fluke, my husband got his first batch of sleep in 3 days. Curled up on the recliner which pulls out to make a mock single bed, he finally got some shut eye. He was a warrior, a trooper, and despite his absolute loathing of being in the hospital and dealing with medical issues such as this, he performed valiantly making sure I was taken care of at every turn.

Since I hadn't gotten around to reading about the last part of my pregnancy or labor and delivery being only 5-6 months pregnant I was not prepared for the next few weeks. Not by a long shot. I had all of the post partum symptoms though they were accelerated. First things first was a few hours after delivery I had my epidural removed as well as my catheter. That was pretty simple. I was then escorted to the bathroom by the nurse. Since my legs had been paralyzed someone had to help me walk and make sure I didn't fall. The nurse also monitors the amount of blood and discharge to note any potential issues. That is fun. She showed me how to create the soothing panty pack. This consisted of some numbing foam on top of a shake and break ice pack that sat like a pad affixed into a disposable panty with some witch hazel pads layered on like lunchmeat for additional comfort. Having someone watch me go to the bathroom was a bit humiliating. I understand the reasoning, my legs were numb and I had just been through a trauma and had a lot of drugs. Subsequent to the epidural I also developed a slight fever. Not good. This was going to potentially keep me in the hospital an extra day. All I wanted to do was go home. Go home and crawl into bed with my dogs and cry. I didn't sleep much, and you don't in the hospital if you didn't know that already, there is always someone coming around to wake you up. In my case the fever meant someone monitoring me every few hours. I will say after the delivery and the epidural and the catheter I really didn't have any pain.

The next morning the doctor on call came in to check me out. He was just darling, it was like George Clooney in ER except he was super tall, coming into my room. I wanted to go home so bad and the nurses kept telling me that because of my fever there was a good chance I was going to have to stay another 24 hours. I also had a fun emotional experience during my short stay. My parents and sister and brother in law came by first thing in the morning after staying with me all day the day before. They brought breakfast and hung out to keep us company. So after my husband got about 4 hours sleep, the first and only in the last 3 days, he called his father. Here is something they don't tell you. The reactions. My husband put his father on speaker phone. His father was living with his girlfriend about 2 miles from the hospital we were at. They didn't come by. They didn't offer sympathy. My husband calls and tries telling his dad that I'm ok, that I had the baby and I was doing fine. My father in law cut him off and said I can't talk now, I'm teeing off. He then hung up. My family, 2 nurses and doctor heard this. My father in law didn't speak to us for a year. That was the last we heard from him. Whether he didn't like dealing with loss or death or what have you, he didn't offer any comfort or even a sorry for your loss. Nothing. It was his 2nd grandchild. He was the first one who was told I was pregnant. That's the reality of being pregnant. Some people are over the moon happy for you, some are jealous, and some are completely ambivalent. A fantastic wonderful and dear friend of mine had given birth the week before up in Los Angeles, and she offered to drive herself and her baby and her mom down to sit with me in hospital and take care of me. She had just had a c-section and that wasn't going to stop her from offering to support me in any way she could.

So after this phone call that still sits very badly with me, the doctor who is tall and handsome looks at me and says, yes a fever will usually keep you here but I think you are fine and we will release you right after lunch. Thank you God like doctor for your kindness. Before we left the social worker visited us again and asked if we needed any counseling or assistance. The hospital Chaplin also came by. He was a character. He prayed with us. He had a big gold pinkie ring on and he smelled like cigarettes. We weren't in a position to turn away anyone who wanted to pray with us. I don't remember a lot of what happened in the hospital for that 36 hours. Or even for the next week. I was sad when I found out the baby had died. I was relieved after I delivered and we were able to kind of leave that situation at the hospital. Not having to hold a funeral was a blessing that I will always be grateful for.

The next month was new ground for me. I bled more than I had anticipated. You are told to abstain for 6 weeks. I bled most of that time. That first week is a killer. I bled everywhere and on everything. My boobs exploded 3 days post delivery. No one warned me about that.   That my body wanted to nurse but there was no baby to feed so my boobs became engorged and insanely painful. Lots of hot showers and massage. I was back to walking a few days later and in the gym the next weekend. It took the full six weeks to start losing any weight. I found that with all of my pregnancies. You have a secret hormone wall that won't allow you to lose more than the hospital weight no matter how hard you work out. Of course as soon as I started shedding that 20+ pounds I had gained I got pregnant again. Another tip after this loss was my mom graciously offered to tell everyone. Since we had passed all of the critical milestones, the 8 week viability and a problem free amnio with perfect results, we had told everyone from our banker to all of our friends and family and co-workers. My mom spent a week letting everyone know that the baby had died. Thank you mom for taking that hit for me. That was one of the biggest favors anyone has over done for me. Not having to relive the pain over and over again trying to explain why I wasn't pregnant anymore to everyone, a true gift my mom gave me, aside from giving birth to me of course. Again, you don't know how people will react. I was shocked and surprised. People who I would consider acquaintances, not close friends overwhelmed me with outpourings of love and support. Cards, flowers, and just warm and well wishes. It was lovely. Then there were some people I was much closer to. My father in law, a friend we had let live with us for the first 4 months of my pregnancy, they disappeared. Didn't call, didn't come see us. Nothing. The hardest was the negative reactions. A few co-workers of mine had some not so nice comments. One said that since I was over 40 there was no way I could carry a baby to term anyway. Another said oh well guess it was God's will. Both hurt in different ways. The over 40 comment was just nasty, and from someone I thought I was very close to, someone I talked to everyday and had helped with numerous personal problems over the years. The God comment wasn't so much about the comment, it just felt hallow. This was a co-worker I saw outside of work, had been to dinner at her house, had worked with her kids to try and help them with some goals in their lives, and I thought we were good friends. The comment just seemed like a blow off. I was glad my mom told every one for me. Six weeks seemed to be the magic number all around. Physically and mentally. It took that long for me to be able to talk about what happened or to tell someone that I lost my baby without bursting into tears. I waited my 6 weeks to have sex, and I was really looking forward to it. I had a period shortly after that. It was weird, not normal since I had been bleeding most of the prior month. I started monitoring my ovulation timing again. I lost baby Grace in May, had my first period at the end of June and was able to get pregnant again in the end of July.

The God comment while it struck me wrong wasn't far off. I wasn't that sad. I was resolved to try again. I had really made peace with the notion that I could not have changed the outcome of baby Grace's existence. Not by being younger or healthier or by living my life different or eating better, nothing I did caused her to die. It just happened. It feels cold to say that. All loses are difficult. I sometimes judge women who have early pregnancy miscarriages and then are destroyed. I had someone try and tell me that their miscarriage was similar to my loss. I didn't agree. Giving birth to a dead baby in the hospital is not the same. I do not have first hand experience but from what I've been told having an early term miscarriage is like having a bad period at home. But I don't discount the emotion of finding out you are pregnant than losing your pregnancy a few weeks later. I guess that is the terminology that defines how I feel about it. Before a certain point, lets say 8 weeks, it's a pregnancy. After that however I feel it's a baby. I had an easy time getting pregnant so maybe that is the disconnect for me. If we had fertility issues I'm sure a miscarriage would rock my world too. We received a card in the mail after our son was born. The hospital was hosting a candle light vigil for the souls that had been lost in the prior year. I still have baby Grace's ultrasounds. They were the prettiest ones I ever got. All of my son's ultrasounds are of his butt and junk and I was able to cut down my medical supervision drastically while pregnant with my daughter and her ultrasound photos are awful. I have to look at the date to see who's pictures are who's. I still have all of the ultrasound pictures in a box. I have her little footprints on a card. I have a sympathy card from the nurses who took care of me that day. Most importantly I have two beautiful healthy happy children that I conceived and gave birth to after this event. That was the best healing. That was what made it better.

11. Everybody Has Something.

I know very few people who have gotten pregnant exactly when they wanted to and without incident. I've had friends who for lack of a steady partner and creeping up the age scale have contracted a sperm bank and had artificial insemination. One woman in particular who after doing IVF with her carefully picked out sperm did get pregnant but the fetus didn't make it and she friend had to have a DNC, that's an abortion if you didn't know. I have another friend who decided to start very late and spent over 10 years and tens of thousands of dollars on fertility treatments. Riding a roller coaster of hormones, weight gain, elation and devastation when she was plagued by miscarriages and then when entering the California foster parent system she was ready to adopt two children who were friends of the family and the mother had severe drug issues and had abused and abandoned the children. After a few months in my friend's care the mom showed back up and was given the children only to abandon them again in a different state. Tragic.

It sounds silly to say I was relieved after our loss. But I was. Relieved that it wasn't something I had done. After the genetic counseling I was relieved that it wasn't because of my age and all of those nasty factors. It was a fluke. A knotted cord. Could have happened to anyone. The whole experience of finding out she was dead and having to deliver it all happened so fast. I found out she was dead on a Friday afternoon and by Saturday evening I had delivered and was home by Sunday. It helped that I didn't feel like anything I did contributed to the loss. That probably helped the most. But having a loss really kills your street credibility with the doctors. Having my son a year later let me be more in control of my medical care for my last pregnancy. He gave me legitimacy that I was a viable mother and had the capability of having healthy babies.

Almost everyone has something. A miscarriage, or two. Trouble getting pregnant when they want to. Or problems during their pregnancy, like gestational diabetes or preeclampsia. Even further down the road, baby stuck in breach or labor that doesn't progress and puts strain on the baby. A million different variables, 99 problems. We had ours in a sense, and I almost felt like we got it out of the way. I mourned, I was devastated, but I carried on and it wasn't even a question with my husband that we would try again. We got a card in the mail for a candlelight vigil being held for the lost babies at our hospital. My husband was furious. Don't forget to pay attention to your husband and his feelings during any loss or bump in the road. It's unrealistic to expect that he feels exactly the same as you or that the same remedies will make him feel better or put him at ease. My husband is highly protective. He doesn't want anyone messing with me or hurting my feelings. He got very angry when that card arrived in the mail. Mostly because he didn't want to drudge up those feelings. What if we hadn't been down the road with a healthy baby already? What if we were having fertility issues and stuck in our grief still? If you get away clean, without a miscarriage or fertility issues you are blessed to the heavens. Most of us, however, have something.

12. I Know All There Is To Know About The Gender Game.

My 2 cents is do everything possible not to find out. I can't tell you the pure joy experienced by the very few women I know who were able to keep the gender a secret during their pregnancy. It's hard. It's a lot of work. Much more so as a higher risk expectant mother. It's almost damn near impossible. Consider it a challenge. A character challenge. Can you do it.? Can your husband do it? Can you make your husband do it? Can you keep you mom at bay for 9 months? That turns it into a giant spy game of guarding secrets. Keeping the information from your mom is actually is harder than dealing with your husband. I'm not talking about the new trend of having a gender reveal party to your friends and family, I'm talking about you and your husband NOT FINDING OUT. Trust me, if he knows you will shortly find out too. I went that route a few times and failed. You husband has to be on board because if one of you knows, you shortly will both know either directly from him or indirectly from someone he told.

Go into ultrasounds deaf dumb and blind. You can tell the technician until the end of time, over and over again that you don't want to know the sex of your baby but there are dozens of clues in little things they say and do. With my son I decided I didn't want to know. At 17 weeks the technician told my husband and I that she could tell us definitively what the gender was. That was enough of a clue for me that it was a boy and if she couldn't see a penis she couldn't tell us definitively at that early of a stage. Thanks. Thanks a lot. The only downside of having a friendly, chatty technician.

There are a lot of challenges that come with parenthood. Self discipline and self control not withstanding. What a better time to start practicing then while you are pregnant. If you can please do not find out. From everything I've heard and read its SO worth it. There is so much cute gender neutral baby décor and clothing out there you don't have to worry. Coming up with multiple names, boy and girl names is not only fun but it prepares if you if you are going to try again. There is nothing more beautiful then having your brand new baby in all white. It's not practical for a second but it's gorgeous and there are years, the rest of your lifetime to get girly clothes and boy clothes and trucks and dolls and all of that. If you can employ the discipline, determination and strength of character it takes to not find out, DO IT. I ran into a neighbor the other day at the grocery store. 8 months pregnant with her second baby. Her mom in tow and she said she didn't find out the first time and she isn't finding out this time either. My question was how do you keep grandma from nagging it out of you since they are the group most determined to get you as much stuff as possible before the baby comes and usually the ones that 'have to know.' Grandma answered that yes it's hard and she wished someone would start a gender neutral baby store on line to make it easier for her. The mystery baby store. We don't know what we are having but we need some stuff to get started. Gray is a trendy neutral color that most younger couples are decorating their homes with. If you are panicked about clothing or anything please keep in mind almost any place that sells baby items will take back unused items. Just don't wash the specific stuff before you go to the hospital. You will be doing a load on DAY 2 so don't stress about doing it all beforehand. White bodysuits are so practical and inexpensive and adorable so just go with that.

Not finding out your baby's gender is a challenge, nay a quest, that is rich with rewards, for those that can nobly go forward blindly. Once you have this amazing wonderful surprise of a lifetime, then you can stock up on colorful boy or girl specific things, that's what the gift cards you get at your baby shower are for anyway. If you can muster the resolve the rewards are so great. I wish I had done it.

13. "We" Are Pregnant Aka Your Husband Is An Idiot.

"Our family" is happily expecting a new member. There is no **WE**. There may be some new situations introduced to your marriage. You may need your husband to be extra loving and supportive. But you are pregnant, not him. Just like "we" are not getting a vasectomy, he is. "We" don't need super plus tampons this month, I do. If it happens directly and solely to your body then you are pregnant, not "we". My husband was along for the ride. I had the bi-polar emotional swings and the gas and the poking and the probing and the tests and the weight gain and the indigestion and the back pain and the swollen ankles. My husband had to deal with a hyper version of me with extra sauce and hormones. My husband was perfection while I was pregnant. My husband played everything right, for me at least. Here is what he did. He told me to eat whatever I wanted during my last pregnancy. Awesome. Having that permission that he wasn't going to not love me if I got really fat I ate everything. Everything and got to the point that in month 8 I was done. I ate what I had wanted to, gorged and indulged every craving, and was over it. He accompanied me to every single appointment he could which was over 95% of them. Being high risk during my second pregnancy that was quite a bit. At least 2 a month for the first few months then they escalated. He didn't overly inject his opinion on anything. He made very social casual conversation with all of the doctors and technicians but never expressed anything other than care and concern for my health and the babies health. He never disclosed or discussed any medical issues with anyone. It wasn't his pregnancy and he acted accordingly. It was his wife's. He was a staunch and seamless supporter of me and my decisions. He was invited to a 'bro' weekend along with various trips while I was late in my pregnancies. Nope can't go. Ridiculous not to be around in case something happens. That's the answer we are going for here. I know a lady who's husband went to Fiji, yes Fiji, for a 2 week long trip when she was 8 months pregnant so he could have a good time before he got 'weighed down" with his 2nd child. She just waddled herself to the bathroom to throw up and focused on taking care of their 8 year old 'special needs' child. You will find that the last month is awful no matter how fit or how happy you are. It's hard. Those last few weeks, no matter how cheery and positive of a person you are you will complain. You will be miserable. So hey husbands, take off to Fiji for a few weeks for a bro-cation. No worries. You work so hard, you deserve it.

We never had a conversation about. I never told my husband my expectations or how I wanted him to act. Rub my feet, be nice, that kind of stuff. My husband made fun of me when I couldn't control my farting and would always make a comment after using the bathroom if I had recently gone. We don't have that type of relationship where my husband would tell people that "we" were pregnant. It's nonsense. The only liberty I will give is with a loss. I do think that is a "we" situation. Yes that is definitely a "we" situation because the loss is shared across the entire family.

One of the first pregnancy support items I bought was a DVD about giving birth. I wasn't going to attend any birthing classes so I thought this was the next best thing. What a joke. It walked through about 6 couples and their different experiences. I learned more watching specials on TLC than I did from this expert birthing video. One thing that left a really bad taste in my mouth was in more than one instance the husband was a staunch and vocal proponent for NOT getting an epidural. That after hours and hours of hard labor as their wives were hitting transition they kept reminding their wives of the decision 'we' had made to have a 'natural' child birth. What the F! Really? "We" don't want any drugs, "we" can tough it out, "we" took birthing classes. No you dumb nut. You sat behind your pregnant wife during class while she practiced her breathing. Uggghhh. I found it so off putting and distasteful and just yuck.

I do appreciate the new age view that men should share equally in the lives of their children. I love that the dads are into it. It's such a change from when my husband and I were kids. I think it's great to see yourself as a family unit right out of the gate and as an experience to be shared as a couple. I think that is wonderful and I am not trying to discourage or make fun of that. My husband is a perfect candidate for a stay at home dad. However I don't expect my husband to equally share in my periods or pregnancy. And seriously guys, have some dignity. Don't end up like those guys are on the EHarmony commercials talking about love and falling in love. We know you have feelings. We know you have a soul. We know you are pumped to be a husband and a dad but really it's not a "We" game it's a "Me" game because as much as you want to share in the experience the bottom line is for your husband it's like going clothing shopping with you. He gets to sit in a chair. He sits a lot. He sits at doctors appointments. He sits during ultrasounds. He sits in the car driving you around to your appointments. He sits in the car when he picks up drive thru fries and a shake for you in the wee hours of the night. He sits in the hospital room. For hours on end. He does get to stand once, during labor, at your shoulders offering words of encouragement but just like when you take him shopping he's not there to give you his truth, his opinion, he is only there to tell you what you want to hear. My husband didn't say a word except after our doctor arrived he said "Dr. Salzetti is here. It's going to be ok" That is the only time I remember him speaking during the birth of my daughter. He recalls that he was panicked until the doctor showed up then he was fine. We want their presence while we go through all of the various stages of pregnancy and all of the appointments etc. The indignity. Pulling your panties and maternity pants back on after an ultrasound and exam. Now I could live without my husband seeing that, especially as I wipe the extra lubricant from my lady parts with the paper table cover. I tried to talk my husband out of coming with me to a few. He insisted. He's a good man. I tried to talk him out of coming to the hospital for the delivery of our last baby and I certainly tried to send him home immediately after. He wasn't budging. We didn't even argue about it. That is the key too. To know when you are necessary and stick to your guns no matter what your hormonally charged wife says. My husband never pissed me off or ruffled my feathers. That is SO A++ in my book. He had a light a social relationship with all of the medical personnel we dealt with. He was aces. Perfect. Present but not pushy. On board but not bossy. "We" were a team, but I was pregnant and having the baby.

14. Finding The Perfect Father.

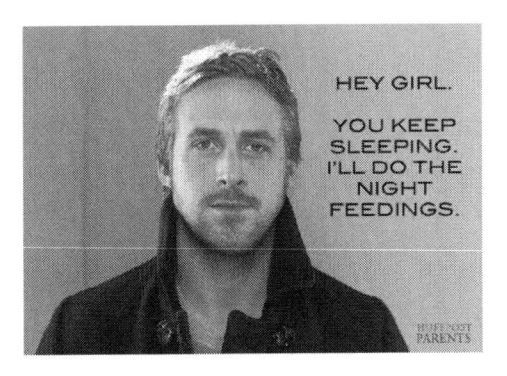

> HEY GIRL.
>
> YOU KEEP SLEEPING. I'LL DO THE NIGHT FEEDINGS.

Is my husband perfect? In my eyes absolutely and he has that daddy gene that is not only ridiculously attractive but it makes your life and your children's life so much better. I guess this is something you need to look at BEFORE you get pregnant, but as it goes men are much different and they mostly become emotionally invested after the baby arrives. Makes sense, since they don't have the little one living inside of them for 9 months.

Now my husband didn't gush over me while I was pregnant. I don't like that stuff and he isn't into it either. He supported me though in a way that was beyond reproach. He was my partner. He stood by me during everything and never once questioned that 6th donut or the fact that I was in the kitchen plowing through a pint of Ben & Jerry's. I felt him and his support always, but his interference or disappointment, never.

My husband is that dad who doesn't have to be asked to pitch in with the kids. He's the dad that doesn't need instructions before you sneak out to get some time to yourself. He's the one the kids are so excited to see at the end of the day and the one they want to tuck them into bed. He's the one that no matter what type of day he has had, and how bad it's been, it all gets shrugged off and shed like snake skin right after he walks in the door and his attention and heart are with his children 100%, well except during college football season, then it's like 90% but he is at home with them in their presence the entire time. I remember a phrase from my childhood, something I saw on TV maybe during a Phil Donahue interview where a man said the best gift he could give his children was to love their mother. I couldn't agree more thought I hit the mother load with having my husband being born with that super dad gene that makes him the most awesome dad on the planet. He's firm but so much fun and he has the respect of not only our kids but our kids friends. They all love him and look up to him as an authority figure as well as a friend and mentor.

At the end of the day you want a partner to share the load like Sam and Frodo in the Lord of the Rings. You are the ring bearer, but he is the one who tries to lighten the load and insure your safety through the journey. He isn't going to break a sweat or get a good workout in walking with you from time to time to help you get some exercise and fresh air, but he does it anyway to keep you company. He wasn't really going to be in the neighborhood that has your favorite bakery but he says he was anyway and he stops by and gets you your favorite treat. He rubs your feet and offers to paint your toes when you can't reach them anymore. This is when those sappy as jewelry commercials get it right, this is the time where your husband needs to become your best friend as well as your protector. If your partner balks at your weight, smell, lack of energy, or any other pregnancy related symptom, but mostly your weight, you my friend have a problem.

15. Naming Your Child.

Don't be a jerk. Seriously. All of your cute trendy names will not hold up in 20 years when your kid starts job hunting after college. I'm cursed with meeting a whole bunch of younger moms in my group that all have what used to be stripper names. Crystal, Amber, all of those elemental names along with the seasons, Sommer, Autumn, coupled with statement names like Destiny sprinkled with tons of Tiffani's and the occasionally city like Paris and Savannah. All used to the standard fare for strippers and porn stars. It's embarrassing. Equally so is naming your child something so specific and so exotic it hinders their progress in life. I say very smugly that my children all have strong classic names. My criteria for choosing a name was the following; what will hold up in 20 years and look good on ESPN, CSPAN, CNN, FNN, etc. Now up at the podium the senator from the great state of California...... Elizabeth Ramirez. Not Harper Brooklyn. Ocean Reign. Jermajesty Jackson. North West. Blue Carter. You get the picture. I am baffled by the trend of naming girls boys names. Again, a lifetime of explaining to teachers, employers, etc. that yes I'm a girl but my parents named me James, Maxwell, etc. Don't burden your child for their ENTIRE LIFE with your foolish choices because it's not about you and your 13 year old wish book dream name. Your desire to be or sound cool amongst your peer group should not dictate a foolish name choice. I can't tell you how many young women I run into in their hopes to aspire to being just like a D list celebrity copy their children's weird names. You don't want to curse your spawn with an albatross around their neck, you want to give them wings to fly. It's about them. And if you want to wait, WAIT. It's not a crime to not find out the gender or name your baby beforehand. If I had the option to not find out what we were having I would have taken it. I tried. It's hard. You don't need those block letters lining the nursery walls a head of time. Your baby can't really see let alone read.

16. Eating Godzilla Style

It took several trips before the lunch shift floor manager at the local Indian food restaurant realized I was pregnant and brought me complimentary lasses, for those that don't know lasses are the Indian version of a yogurt smoothie that take the edge off of the spiciness of most Indian foods. I think she just thought I was fat while eating 6 plates of food with tons of mint chutney and tamarind sweet sauce piling it in my mouth with a basket full of fresh garlic nan bread. Maybe she thought I prepping for a competitive eating contest. I could give old Joey Chestnut a run for his money at the Nathan's 4th of July Hot Dog Eating Contest, well if hot dogs weren't on the 'do not eat' list. The guy who holds the ice cream eating record is nicknamed 'deep dish.' GTFO. Then call me pregnant Jabba the Hut and bring on the food.

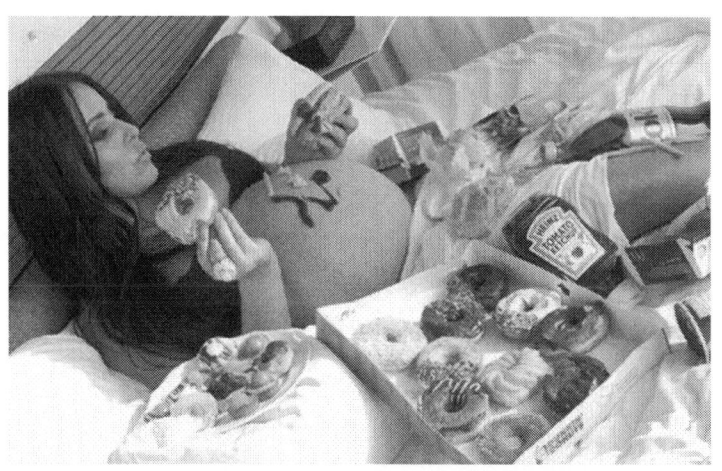

Unkonwn Source for this photo but it's AWESOME

While pregnant I ate everything. Cookies, cake, cupcakes, candy bars, burgers, fries, you name it I ate it. The mystique of it lost its luster around month 8 of my last pregnancy but I can tell you it made me really happy. When you feel nauseous or sick or tired or blah a milkshake can do wonders. Food while pregnant becomes your only vice since smoking, drinking, and you aren't Courtney Love so heroin and crack are no no's. You have stress, you are tired, you have anxiety, and ice cream can help. I don't regret anything I ate. Not a thing. My ability to lose weight after my last baby is a black hole. I gained too much and created some pretty bad daily eating habits especially involving sweets and now I can't get those last 20 pounds off. Oh well. I was happy. Content. Fat and pregnant. No better feeling in the world than eating and napping while cooking a little baby in your belly. I've read studies that suggest that you eat more junk food when you don't get enough sleep. For me that could not be more true. My ability to make better choices goes downhill the more tired I am. I didn't sleep much during my last pregnancy. I had molten lava heart burn and acid reflux that could not be quenched. It was rough and ice cream and cake made it better. I'm sure fruit smoothies and low fat yogurt would have helped to but, ehh not as fun.

I was obsessed with food. With lists of food. With shows about food. All things food. In the morning I would think about what I was going to eat that day and at night I would fantasize about what I was going to eat in the morning. I would read recipes just to think about what the food must taste like. Look at pictures of food. I have a natural sweet tooth so my pregnancy cravings moved me into eating whole cakes. I learned to bake so I could eat cake and cupcakes. I made cookies. I made lemon bars. Food TV was like porn to me. I learned to make sauces. Sauces. Like border line grown up cooking.

Truthfully in the swamp of my eating habits while pregnant I stayed away from the taboo foods like hotdogs, lunchmeat, sushi, etc. I took a pre-natal vitamin daily. In fact I'd taken a pre-natal vitamin daily for the last 4 years. Take them to prepare, take them while pregnant, take them while nursing, take them to prepare for the next pregnancy, etc. I peed bright yellow for half a decade. I did not take a holistic approach to my eating however. I didn't focus on antioxidants or whole foods. I don't regret that. Not for a second. If I had been in my twenties and having a whole mess of kids I would have done one very sloppy pregnancy where I ate what I wanted and rested a lot. Followed by a very clean pregnancy of good eating and fitness. In my 40's really I was like screw that. While pregnant with my son I was so riddled with anxiety and stress having just had a loss and being put on restricted activity that I wasn't a total food monster but I wasn't a good hipster granola girl either. I kept my gym membership for a few months and did pre-natal yoga pretty regularly. By the time I was pregnant with my daughter which I knew was going to be my last pregnancy ever, the flood gates on my eating were removed. I did my yoga until about 7 ½ months then I was too tired and in too much pain to go anymore. One of the last classes I went to I ate 5 pieces of pizza before hand and spent the entire session with my butt tensed up so I wouldn't fart and peel the paint off of the walls. Yeah I ate. I chased after a toddler, I was so sick the whole time. Crazy magma quality acid indigestion to the point where I needed industrial prescription antacids. For some reason I survived a few Indian buffets but could not eat Mexican food without really regretting it for a day or two. My throat would be backed up with Alien acid.

My favorite pregnancy foods.

LilDeb4Life Cold Little Debbie's Swiss Cake Rolls. I refrigerated mine for maximum yumminess. Then I would slowly unroll them when I wasn't eating them like sushi and shoving the whole thing in my mouth. Are you kidding? Heaven.

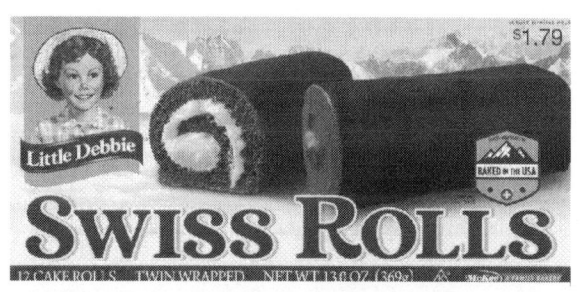

Little Debbie Swiss Cake Rolls, McKee Foods Inc.

@ *TikiNanChutneyOhMy!!!* Indian Buffet with a Mango Lasse. Plateful upon plateful of exotic goodness. The spices weaving a symphony in my nose and on my tongue. As close to heaven as you can get using hot fresh garlic nan as a scoop with extra mint and sweet chutney on top. Sweet, smooth, creamy, soothing, and just plain delicious. Milk shakes have nothing on a lasse treat plus it helps that 6th plate of Indian food go down so much smoother.

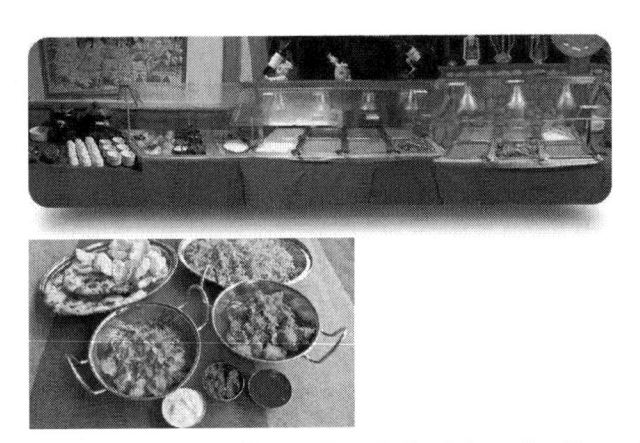

All you can eat Indian Food buffet at Indian Princess San Marcos, CA

CHeezBurgParadize Plain Cheeseburger and Fries. Don't need mustard, ketchup or onions. Just give me meat and cheese and let me soak in that grease and saltiness. Save the ketchup for my fries. And supersize that bitch will ya? I'm eating for two!!! Back off while I'm eating and if you decide to get all HamBurglar on me and try to steal my fries I will cut you. You will bleed. I will mix your blood with ketchup and eat that too. Don't touch my fries.

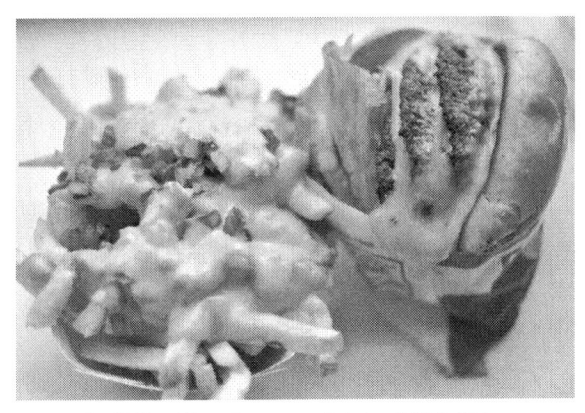

In-N-Out Cheeseburger and Animal Style Fries

#CAKE&CAKE Anything Cake. Cake mix at my grocery store would go on sale for $1 and frosting $2. I was baking cakes and cupcakes every few weeks and I could eat a dozen cupcakes and a can of frosting in a sitting. Too sweet you say? Well I also learned how to make my own simple powdered sugar frosting to take that

super artificial taste out. The worlds' most favorite cake man, our boy Duff Goldman (or Duffy as his mom calls him) says you cut the cupcake in ½ and make it like a sandwich with the frosting in the middle. Preach Duff preach. I'm there. I'm all over it.

@ ChoCoHolllick!! Anything chocolate. That was me and as you can tell I already had a propensity for sweets before I got pregnant. On an eating level being pregnant is like being stoned. Your cravings are serious, weird, and oddly specific. Skinny ladies will tell you it's your body and your baby letting you know what you need. Hogwash, well mostly hogwash. Similar to being stoned your senses are in overdrive. The pregnancy hormones give you a crime dog McGruff caliber nose which enhances the flavor of everything. Plus you've given up all of your vices so the food is all you got. Trader Joes sells some killer truffles and Hershey symphony bars have toffee bits and the end all of easy to purchase chocolate Dove has milk, dark, all types of different easy to consume bags of individually wrapped chocolates. An entire bag in one sitting? HELL YES!

@ SmellsLikeTeenFeet?!? Pepsi. Can't stomach it any other time but the hormones raging through my system make it crave worthy. Not coke. Not Mr. Cola. Pepsi. Ice cold please. Thank you.

 # TheRealGreenSmoothie Shamrock Shake. It's all about the timing here. I'm not saying you should plan your pregnancy around the McDonald's menu offerings, McRib says what?? But I'm just saying a Shamrock Shake hits the spot.

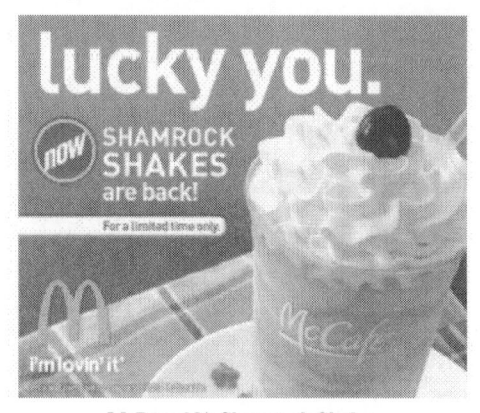

McDonald/s Shamrock Shake

#ButIt'sHealthy Pistachio muffins and all forms of not so good for you snacks and treats that you buy at the healthier grocery store under the pretense that it must be good for you because it's available at the healthier grocery store. I hope you know it's a crock of nonsense. It's all the same as muffins you buy at the regular store. About 500 calories each you might was well have a cupcake. That's what a muffin is a breakfast cupcake and lord help you if you get the chocolate chocolate chip. IT's a CUPCAKE – just ask Duff. He'll tell you.

@ *SideORanch* Ranch dressing with and on everything. No further explanation needed. Especially hot fries then occasionally a salad when you want to feel 'healthy.'

#LoveItButtItDoesn'tLoveMe Mexican food. My friend. My foe. My love. My enemy. Doesn't mix well with earth shattering volcanic heartburn. Carne Asada burrito with guac and a side of carrots. Love. Doesn't love me. I had to give it up month 6 on the last pregnancy. It's like when I gave up drinking in my early 30's. The next day was so much worse than any joy received from the consumption. Bummer.

@ *IceColdDrPepperHere!* There is nothing nothing like an ice cold soda. Be careful with the caffeine but seriously it makes you feel so good. The sugar, the caffeine and the ice cold goodness. I found myself overheating in a minute while I was pregnant and having a hell of a time cooling down. Ice cold soda fixes so many problems, from your stomach to your fatigue, from a headache to helping you cool down from the inside. Not a watered down fast food soda, but an actual from a can, or better yet from a bottle. They have real Coke a Cola in bottles made with real sugar bottled in Mexico at the Home Depot's here in San Diego. Better than sex.

DQBlizzardLUVIT Dairy Queen in your friend when you are pregnant. For real. Everything is not only solid, and that's saying a lot from someone who hasn't consumed fast food in quite a long time, but the menu is ideal for you when you are in the knocked up way. It's simple, not spicy, and coats your stomach. One of the

hurdles I found is that the more my stomach felt out of whack or I had a slight headache the floodgates would open and I'd want to eat everything in sight just to get it to stop. Ice cream, shakes, check check. Simple burgers and chicken with Texas toast. Double check. Their fries are ok. If that's your thing hit up Carl's Jr. or Jack n the Box for some serious criss cut fries or even an In and Out. But as far as wanting to eat a decent pregnancy gluttonous meal, the DQ has it going on. If I had been a competitive eater, which I should have attempted while pregnant, I would have a shirt filled with sponsors and my largest would be DQ.

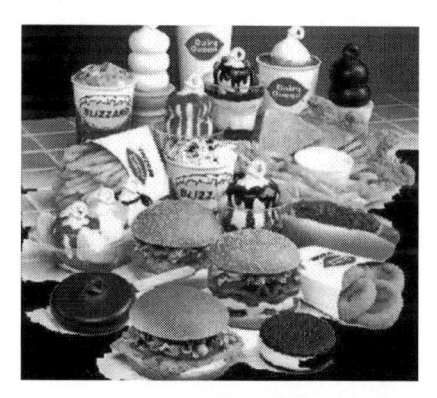

Dairy Queen DQ™

Coming back from a pre-natal exam once I stopped at McDonalds. I got a Shamrock shake and a plain quarter pounder with cheese. Heaven. I would bake a cake during the day so I would have something to snack on. Every day I found myself wanting sweets and I would stop for a candy bar at CVS on the way home from work and end up with chips, candy, chocolate bars, and ice cream. My husband took me to Five Guys a few times while I was pregnant. If you've ever been there a large fry should be called a heart attack special because it's so frickin big. I would eat one with very little help from the rest of my crew and about 5 of those paper cup things filled with ketchup. Their burgers are good. Like Wendy's original burger good. When Wendy's actually used to cook their burgers to order instead of microwaving them their motto was something like so juicy you need a napkin. And they were. They used to drip grease like a homemade backyard burger with low quality high fat ground beef. Speaking of back yard grill block BBQ burgers Diary Queen has an exceptional offering. There were days I would get their double burger, fries, and a blizzard. Maybe a banana pie blizzard or something seasonal. They also have a very decent chicken fingers basket with fries and Texas toast. Yum. Top that with a banana split and you are gold. Back in my party days I used to eat at Jack n the Box. Mostly because they were one of the few drive thru's in my area that stayed open late. Sounds weird but they have the BEST eggrolls. And taquitos. I don't know why they are so good but if you have never tried them you should. Let's not get so sidetracked with burgers and fries that we lose that other American staple, pizza. I could eat a whole pizza by myself, it was sick. The worst was eating pizza before yoga class. Pizza with it's cheese and sauce would ignite my roaring acid reflux and indigestion into a whole different league. Sticking with Italian a nice Italian cheesecake, a meatball or an eggplant parmesan sub would do the trick too. Now I've met ladies who claim that during their pregnancy they craved fruit and vegetables. I did too. In the enormity of the daily consumption I actually had a prenatal vitamin and a well rounded meal in there but the rest was all garbage. BTW my kids came out just fine and my dozens of donuts et. al did not effect them one iota. So belly up to the buffet. It's a celebration. Time to eat.

17. Yoga. Not Just For Hipsters And Old Ladies.

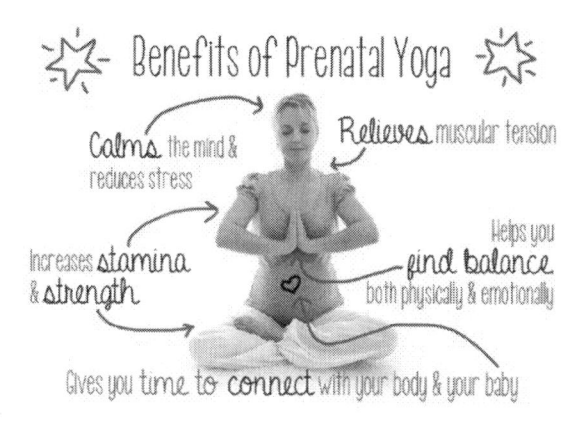

Benefits of Prenatal Yoga

- Calms the mind & reduces stress
- Relieves muscular tension
- Increases stamina & strength
- Helps you find balance both physically & emotionally
- Gives you time to connect with your body & your baby

Image from One Down Dog.com

So I'm in class which a bunch of very new age, eco friendly, Millennial women. Those ladies who are stocking up on their antioxidants and only eating healthy foods. Yeah well we are all gaining weight regardless. I tried endlessly to entice them to go to Popeye's Chicken or the donut shop with me after class. No takers. Seriously ladies WE are all gaining weight regardless, and a little treat will make you feel better. All within driving and smelling distance of the place we do our yoga is not only Popeye's and Yum Yum Donuts, but an In and Out, Asian Buffet and a Roberto's Taco Shop. It's a scientific fact if you eat a bunch of crap and milk shakes and junk food while you are pregnant you feel so so much better than if you eat a low fat, high protein, organic food healthy calorie counting diet.

Pre-natal yoga is a God send. Everyone should do it even if you've never done yoga before. It helps on so many different levels. There are breathing exercises, relaxation, flexibility and core strengthening. You first start the class breathing. Sounds silly but a skill you are going to need later. Breathing is a central core theme of delivery. Both breathing out and holding your breath. There are breathing exercises where you breathe in through your nose, and out through your mouth. Some you make a low humming noise, my instructor called it bee breathing. You need it later so pay attention. Learning to extend your inhales and exhales will help during delivery. Then there is your core, you know you can't do sit ups while pregnant, bummer, but you still need those muscles later to deliver, dilemma. Keeping your core as strong as possible through yoga practice is essential. It is invaluable. Do it. It will help. Finally gaining a lot of weight, for some ladies for the first time gaining that much that quickly, coupled with aches and pains takes your flexibility down several notches. Think about your knees pinned back behind your ears during delivery and you will soon realize while maintaining some of that limberness is a task worth undertaking.

Not to be discounted, especially if you already have a few kids at home, is getting out of the house for a few hours a week to be with other pregnant ladies. Being in a group of 10-20 mother's to be brings a solidarity and a unity of purpose. It's a comfort being with a group of women going through the exact same thing you are. Of course there are always comparisons. Some of these bitches bend like yogi masters with their giant baby bellies but skinny legs and sick flexibility. Some ladies were bigger like me and just trying to get through the classes. Some were older, some younger, some had tons of kids, for some it was their first.

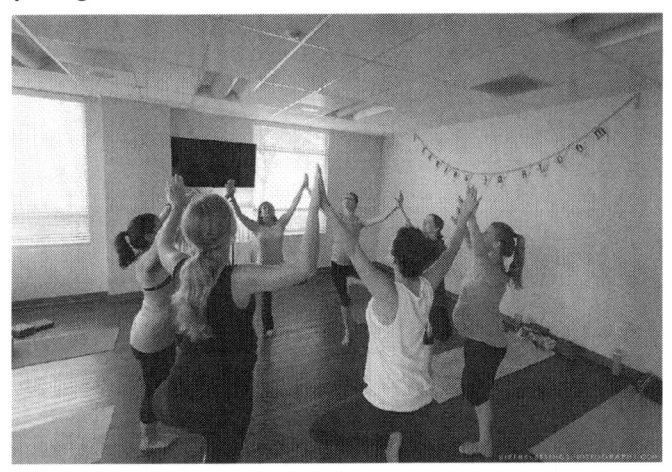

Photo from YogaJanda

So again first you do some breathing exercises, then several different poses and positions in sequence, then is the best part. Corpse pose. Doesn't sound fun but it's the best. You lay on your back and relax your arms and legs and in our class the instructor gave us an eye pillow sprayed with lemongrass scent and you lay down and relax and clear your mind for about 5 minutes to soothing music. It's an hour well spent by all accounts and not only readies your body but your mind. I credit doing yoga with the relative ease of my deliveries. I felt like my stomach muscles were in decent enough shape to push effectively, as well as the exercises that loosened up my pelvis, those help a lot. Your old pelvic girdle takes a beating and practicing yoga helps you maintain a suppleness in that region.

The downsides are going with indigestion or gas. I struggled several times not to let one rip or throw up during class. There hit a point where my acid indigestion was so extreme that I thought I was going to breathe fire during a downward dog. My instructor was the bomb, and didn't mind too much when we were in compromising position that I'd pipe in about how I had recently been in that pose and had may have actually conceived while doing it. There are some suggestive hip gyrating, pelvis thrusting on all fours like you are being pounded on the stairs moves going on. All to open up and add suppleness in your pelvic region. You need that familiarity with the muscles down there in order to push and to push properly. I find to this day I try to stretch and do yoga on a daily basis. It's a good healthy routine to get into. Where I live they've even tried putting yoga in the schools as part of PE and helping kids calm down and focus. Of course there are some wonderful people who claim that yoga is too religious and have had it subsequently banned but it was a good idea. Doing yoga is never bad and every time you do it its like money in the bank. Really unless you are one of those ladies weight lifting and running marathons while pregnant, it's one of the best most consistent and even strenuous exercises to do while pregnant. Can't hurt, always helps. There is nothing like stretching to release tension and teaching kids how to breathe and focus is always a very good thing.

18. Basic Whining And Complaints.

There are a myriad of different physical manifestations of your pregnancy. Nesting, that one is cool. Right before baby comes you are overwhelmed with a compulsion to clean, and I mean dig into corners, rip out the window screens, bleach the bathtub straight up gangster clean your house and set up the nursery. The pregnancy glow, long nails and shiny hair. Wonderful. However, no one likes a skinny pregnant bitch who is happy and having a problem free pregnancy. For the rest of us, the fun has just started.

Butt Sweat: I can't tell you how many times you are going to have to take your clothes off and lay naked on the wax paper exam table with a paper towel over you while someone sticks something inside you. So your sweaty butt will stick to and rip the paper when you get up as you want to wipe because you are gushing with lube. Your husband will greatly enjoy this sexy display. I can't tell you how many people will see you fat, hairy and naked so check your dignity at the door. Tests, exams, inspections with gloves and lots of lube. Tubes of it. You will be sweaty, sticky and stinky. Welcome to the pleasure dome.

I stink: I can tell you for 8 of the 9 months I stunk. Your nose kicks into super TSA drug dog smelling realms and I stunk. Are you kidding? You will have the olfactory capability of a bloodhound. In my case I still have most of that heightened sense to this day. I smelled like pee. I could smell my stinky feet. I could smell everything I would walk into a room and announce "it smells like farts in here." My husband is giving me an honorary PhD in bodily fluid scent detection. Between my stinky, sweaty, flatulent self and my husband the kids and the dogs, I didn't get a break for a single second during my pregnancy from overwhelmingly foul scents that made me wretch.

Hormones: One of the first things my yoga teacher cautioned us about was watching baby shows on TLC. "I Didn't Know I Was Pregnant," "A Baby Story", all of that stuff. The movie "Juno" is a special tear jerker. I broke down while watching "War Horse," I mean I completely and utterly lost it and had to turn it off when the horse was in trouble. My hormones and emotions took over and I was hysterical. The cliché is true that you will start crying at car commercials and all types of sappy stuff which is especially jarring if you are not a sappy person. You will wildly swing while pregnant, up down and sideways. Get ready for the ride.

The worst of you: My husband heard me fart, burp, and panic when I peed on myself. Any illusions that I was a beautiful and dainty flower were shattered the first time I actually peed on myself in front of him and fell asleep on the sofa, drooling, snoring, only to be woken by the explosion of my own farts while my husband was awkwardly starting at me, as if to say what da heck was dat?

Hot topic discussions. I'm not a fan of discussing any of these issues. Poop. Periods. Blood. But having a baby forces your to deal with all of these head on. I had poops while pregnant that smelled worse than my husband's. Every doctor's visit that question hits, when was your last period. There is blood everywhere after delivery and for weeks to come. There is a lot of anxiety and pressure for your first poop after delivery. You will be given Colace. Buy some for at home too. It helps. The meds, stress, et. al can clog you up and the last thing you want to do is strain after delivery. Your parts are beat up enough and you don't want the fear of popping your stitches. You will talk about all of these fun body manifestations with doctors, nurses, your curious friends and family. It's crazy.

Do these pants make me look fat? I'm actively making the case for yoga pants and a zip hoodie. Now I wanted to be one of those cute pregnant women. Pretty dresses and flowy tops. Walking with my husband when he gets home from work in the early evening to get in some exercise together in a cute athleisure outfit with a barely there belly where from behind you wouldn't even realize I was 8 months pregnant. Yeah, not so much. Didn't happen. High-waisted compression yoga pants from the Old Navy, a stretch v neck t-shirt and a hoodie became my pregnancy uniform, which I then promoted to my everyday mommy uniform too.

Medicine: My first pregnancy I took nothing. It only last 6 months but I didn't take anything. Second pregnancy cut way down on caffeine but didn't take other meds. I felt like a superhero, the surging hormones making me stronger, better, faster, well not faster but you get the picture. Third pregnancy oh my gosh. Tylenol and prescription strength antacids. It scared me to take so much medicine, more than I had taken collectively in the past 20 years, but it had to be done. I could not function with the heartburn, I couldn't even walk down the stairs, I couldn't lay down, I couldn't sleep. Also there was no way I could let my fevers fester for fear for the baby inside me having a problem. I ran through a bottle of Tylenol and 4 months of prescription antacids. I was a disaster to the point where my husband told me on more than once occasion that this should be my last pregnancy. I felt like I could do it but man it was hard. The physical ailments piled up day after day. I didn't feel them hit me all at once but at the end I was barely functional.

All around if you are having a mild pregnancy celebrate that and enjoy that you are feeling well because there are a lot of women out there who are absolutely miserable, on their knees praying to the toilet gods, bowels backed up to before the Berlin Wall came down, who can't eat, sleep, walk or talk normally for the duration. Having other children changes your pregnancy, at least it did for me. Having a toddler during my last pregnancy changed up the fact that when I felt like shredded dog poop I couldn't check out for a few hours and run out for a milkshake and take a nap. I had a million chores to do and another little person to take care of. I didn't realize how bad of shape my body was in until about 15 minutes after I had my little girl and I finally felt better. The weight off of my back, gone. The pressure on my chest that made me labor to breathe, gone. The Scorch Trial level heartburn that had plagued me for months, gone. The chronic aches and pains in my joints, gone. All I felt was stitches in my butt, and that was about it. A wave sweeps over you especially after a drug free labor where your body resets its pain thresholds and all of the little stuff kind of evaporates. I can tell you almost 2 years post delivery with my last the small aches and pains are finally creeping in but

I'm also almost 48 years old and my body has been through a lot over the last 5 years. I feel those neck aches, and ankle stiffness, but it's very recent. My mental outlook on what I could endure has changed dramatically. I wasn't a wuss before, but I rarely pushed myself and would often take an easy or lazy route out of things. While I'm working out now I know I can push extra hard or do an extra set and I'll be ok. Shooting that last baby out of my crotch absolutely shifted that.

19. The Fear is Real and the Anxiety Overwhelming.

I was scared. Scared to death. Scared for a year straight. I was terrified at every blood draw, every ultrasound, the thought of every needle and every test. While pregnant with my son there was not a single day that I didn't think he was going to die inside me. Every kick count was agony. He didn't kick that hard and every day I thought I was going to have to go down to the ER and be monitored and I would be told he was dead. The litany of appointments where the worst case scenarios are served up on a silver platter for your consumption, so that you are "informed" and the medical practice covers their butts. No one ever sat down and read me a list of the wonderful things that would come with having a baby, just the dismal prospects of having a child that would have some malformation or deformity and if I got away clean physically the chances that my kids would be autistic or have learning disabilities based sole on my age were mind numbing. Actually having a baby, taking care of the baby, that part didn't shake me one bit. It was the medical procedures that got me. The thought of my son being circumcised and having part of his penis cut off. His penis!?! Are you kidding me? Stitches up and down my pussy. Litacain shots on the outer lips of my vagina and my taint. Get out of here! A giant needle going into my stomach and a few months down the road another one going into my spine. My flipping spine. Oh my god. I'm having sweats and anxiety just thinking about it again. My heart is racing. That then reminds me of all of the monitors and probes.

Your body is a vessel, a chamber for growing this human being and it's being tossed around like an old car that needs a tune up. I had a great doctor and great teams and there is still some inhumane stuff that goes down that everyone in the baby birthing profession sees as standard practice but it's painful and scary and the first time I went through all of it I was absolutely terrified. I did my best to refocus myself. When I was at my worst, my most frightened I remembered a few times in my life where being scared and tense during medical procedures was not helpful. Stupidly I had gum surgery eons ago done in 2 parts. The first ½ I had done I was petrified because they keep you awake for it and just numb the area, sound familiar. I was so tense and uptight that it hampered my recovery and increased my pain levels. For the second half since I knew what to expect I was more relaxed, I took better care of myself afterwards and I did everything I could to calm myself down before and during the procedure. I did the same with being pregnant. I would see the phlebotomist prepping 6 vials and a butterfly needle to draw blood from me. My eyes felt like they were bulging out of my head and I would begin to speed up and get panicked. I would try and project myself someplace else. I would engage in mindless chit chat. I would remind myself that everyone who's had a baby has had to go through this. Well everyone with insurance who chooses to go through the traditional doing it with a doctor route. That no one was there to hurt me and that they knew what they were doing. That was the hardest part to convince myself of actually was that the person on the other end of the needle, the probe, etc. knew what they were doing.

Anesthesiologist, pretty much had no choice but to trust that person. I had 2 epidurals, one to deliver the baby who was already gone and the other for my son. The one for my son went in crooked and came out crooked. What? I knew I was having contractions and I so wanted my husband there but he had gone to grab a cup of coffee because he didn't realize it was all going to happen so quickly so the nurse had to hold my hand during that pleasantry. With an epidural unfortunately goes a catheter. Umm no thank you. The cliché of breathe, just breathe does work in all of these cases. When you are scared out of your mind, terrified beyond all bounds, breathing in and out just to get your mind focused and to calm yourself down. Think back to your yoga practice, calm down and breath and let yourself float on a cloud and project your thoughts elsewhere. I projected myself into the future, what my baby would feel like in my arms, smell like, look like when he looked up at me.

I was tense and anxious for so long I can't remember what it's like to be relaxed. The last time I was truly relaxed and was free of crippling fear was during a massage before I got pregnant. The stress of trying to get pregnant, the anxiety of being pregnant, the outright freak me out fear of delivery, kept me on the edge for over a year. The next level is after the baby comes. Oh my God is he breathing? Am I going to drop him? What if I hurt him? That fear comes in tsunami waves crushing your psyche. It can really get to you, all of it, if you let it. Do your best to relax, have your partner help you ease some of your anxiety by distracting you, making you laugh. Take your mind off of things and center your core by keeping your eyes on the prize. A beautiful brand spanking new baby that is all yours. All of the tests, poking and prodding will be long over at the moment you have that little one in your arms and start your new life together.

III: Having A Baby: OMG Is This For Real?

20. Packing For The Hospital.

Don't overcomplicate things. One of the small joys in life is finding that perfect take home outfit for your baby. I shopped for months looking for that one memorable outfit that would look amazing on my brand new, pure as driven snow, bundle of joy. It's so much fun to have this new little person to dress and shop for. That first outfit however, it's a bit overrated. Not in how happy it makes you finding it, which is a joy to the heavens, but in how it actually fits and how your baby will look in it and you aren't going to get that real perfect going home photograph straight out of the gate. You really don't know until you have that little one what body type they are, small, lean, long, chubby, bigger, you just have no idea and all of the ultrasounds and measurements in the world won't help you. I had cute as hell track suits for both my kids. For my son a size 0-3 month with a football on it. Adorable. With my daughter a white terry suit with a pink giraffe. I had back up outfits too. With hats and blankets and jackets. Just a onesie is fine. If you want to dress baby up for pics, sometimes naked is best for those first pics or even one of your lovely baby blankets because the clothes just don't fit well.

Having said all of that, the last thing you want as you are trying to hustle out of the hospital with your brand new baby is to spend time shit shuffling and going through bags to make sure you have everything you brought. You will NOT want to go back to the hospital to retrieve anything later, you will be far too busy. So don't bring too much and don't bring things that are completely unnecessary. I read dozens of pregnancy books that had the check list for what to bring to the hospital and they were pages upon pages long. It's not Club Med here, and anything you might forget someone can bring for you or you can send your husband out to buy, I promise. Less is more. For sure.

There are some basic categories you need to cover here:

1) **BABY**

    a) **Going home outfit.** A few outfits in a few different sizes if that's the experience you want. I would pack one size zero, one 0-3 month, one newborn size. The different brands cut clothes differently and the size ranges all vary all over the place. It's worse than buying jeans. All of my careful planning across both of my babies and spending months finding and picking out that perfect take home outfit were for naught. Neither fit right, if at all. Your baby will be bigger or smaller than the original outfit you picked out so bring more than one if that is important to you. If not just a plain onesie, maybe a long sleeved one, The simple white Carters ones are awesome for this. Your baby is brand new and white just sets that off so nicely for a boy or a girl. Bring the outfits if you must, I packed mine in Ziploc bags, and it is fun trying them on but as mentioned you don't always get the results you were looking for. Also please keep in mind I live in San Diego, so if you need extra blankets or jackets, just plan for how much your baby is going to be exposed to the cold on the way home.

    b) **A blanket.** A thin cotton blanket and a thicker warm blanket for the car ride.

    c) You might want a **support pillow** for your car seat to help keep baby's neck stable.

    d) **That's really all you need.** The hospital will provide diapers and wipes and a suction bulb for nose and mouth.

2) **YOU – aka The New Mommy** ☺

    a) **Shoes.** Flip flop, slip on shoes, or slippers. The floors of the hospital have more germs and nastiness than the grotto spa at the Playboy Mansion and I've been there, the foam that comes off that thing is insane and resembles a bacteria infested primordial ooze. Always wear something on your feet. Anything that's easy to get on and off, maybe even disposable, and there is a good chance your feet could be swollen so super comfy. You want to disinfect the bottom of your shoes with alcohol when you get home and you don't want your shoes touching anything that is going to touch you or the baby. It's disgustingness at the highest of levels.

    b) **Ziploc bags.** To help you organize things. You will have a boat of supplies to take home. You need about ½ dozen bags just to keep everything organized and separate. You will have some extras if you pack your toiletries in a few. Our hospital provided one plastic see through tote bag and I used that for my dirty clothes which you definitely want to keep away from your baby items as well as your personal feminine items.

    c) **Bathroom items.** Biggest category. What works for you. If you like dry Shampoo, bring it. I find it seriously drying but you might like it. Hair Brush. Hair ties. Make up. Wipes for your face. Hand sanitizer. Lip balm. Lotion. Toothbrush. Toothpaste. Mouth wash. You are going to feel so NASTY. Dirty. Dingy. Covered in layers of gunk and goo. It is Ghostbusters and yes you did get SLIMED. You want something smooth that smells nice to counterbalance just how disgusting it all is. Wipes and lotion and lip balm will go a long way towards that end. Alcohol wipes too. The cleaner the better. Also some nipple cream. I don't remember the hospital providing that.

    d) **Going home outfit.** Simple and comfortable. You will have a LOT going on in your lady regions. Between stitches, soreness, giant pads, ice packs, all of that the bulk in your pants is enormous making yoga pants a hit or miss option actually. You might want a sundress or something equivalent with some capri yoga pants and granny panties underneath to hold all of the pads and packs in place. You'll want maximum coverage, padding and security down there. Layers on top, maybe a tank and a hoodie depending on the weather. I did yoga pants the first time and realized I had such a load in the back of my pants it was frightfully unattractive. I ended up tying a sweatshirt around my waist because I was embarrassed. A long black stretchy skirt works to. You are going from the room to the car then in the house. While it might feel like Fashion Week in New York, it's not. Just aim to look decent and you will be fine as no one you encounter will be focusing on you, all of the attention is on the star of the day, your new baby.

 e) **Odds and ends.** Charger for your phone. Cash. Candy for the nurses. I brought Dove chocolates. Yum.

 f) **Clothes for the hospital.** Most places won't let you bring your own hospital gown though they sell them for about $20 each on Amazon. Hospital gowns are awful and nasty. They are rough and ugly. I didn't have a choice but to wear one for delivery so that first picture is with that gown. Of course you can bring your own clothes for after that but with my son I will tell you I went through 8 gowns in less than 2 days, covered in blood and urine. You might want a nursing bra though I found them useless as you are always either trying to nurse or do skin on skin so being naked under the gown is the best option.

 g) **Information.** Medical insurance of course. Bring your card. They need to photocopy it. Our hospital sent a form in advance for you to fill out and since I went to the hospital in our network my records were easy to access. You are also going to have to fill out some essential forms for your little one like the application for their social security card and their birth certificate. You will need your name and social, your husband's name and social and both of your parents full legal names. Make yourself a file on your phone with pictures of these essential documents and details that will be hard to recall after giving birth and all of the other stress that goes with having a brand new baby.

 h) **Leave the things you don't need AT HOME.** You will be home before you know it. The hospital isn't the place to dilly dally. It's all a blur. Aside from a few pics and visitors you don't need to be dolled up. Its harder to wrangle the unnecessary items when you are in the mad rush to leave and trust me once you are told you can leave it's all you want to do is get out as quickly as you can. With the discharge instructions, how to take care of you, how to take care of your baby, signing releases, grabbing all of the diapers and baby items, grabbing all of the pads and items to help you with your bleeding, the last last last thing you will want to do is figure out where all of your extra shoes and second make up bag is.

 i) You can **BUY** or have your husband or friends bring you things you need. You probably won't, but it's an option. Case in point. With our daughter, who was our second baby, my husband packed nothing for himself. He assumed he would want to go home and relieve my parents who were taking care of our toddler son but he didn't. He didn't leave the hospital except to grab a bite and grab some clothes at the mall down the street. He bought himself some underwear, a shirt and shorts. Done and done. Men simplify things and I like it.

21. It Just Got Real Round 1.   Full Moon On Friday The 13th.

The first time I went into labor it was pretty mild at the onset. For some reason I was more afraid to be in false labor and be turned away from the hospital. I don't know why. I mean really afraid of being judged or labeled or someone thinking I was stupid for going to the hospital before I was actually ready. Now I had a labor plan. Everyone does. The problem is the people who have the plan and want everyone to stick to it. Good luck with that. I've heard of 3-4 page plans being printed out and handed out at the hospital. Ummmm yeah. My plan was more along the lines of a wish list really. I was over 40 so there was no way I wasn't going to the hospital. Not for me but for the baby. I also didn't want to be at the hospital laboring for an ungodly amount of time. Finally I wanted to do everything I could to avoid a c-section. With what I call modified and realistic expectations I got all of my wishes.

I started laboring on a Thursday night. I wasn't sure if it was real. Went to bed but was up by 4am. Took a very long shower, shaved, finished packing my hospital bag with my daily necessities like my contacts and glasses and toothbrush. Around 9am I was having contractions that were stopping me in my tracks. My stepdaughter was home with us and I didn't want her to see me in pain so I'd step into the closet or turn away. I called my doctor's office around 10am to ask if I should wait to come in that day, I had a 1pm appointment, or go to the hospital The litmus testing for going to the hospital is called **511. Contractions 5 minutes apart, lasting 1 minute in duration, steady for 1 hour**. By 12:30 I had a contraction in the kitchen that brought me to my knees. My husband said that I was a tough person and if that was happening I was probably in labor. Off to the hospital we went. Now my husband got a nervous stomach so we had to stop so he could go to the bathroom. It was a Friday the 13th. It was a full moon. It was raining. I'm sitting in the parking lot calling and texting my friends and family saying we are on the way to the hospital and here come my contractions. For the rest of the car ride they were about 2-3 minutes apart. I was grabbing onto the "oh shit" handle and hoping and praying to not have the baby in the car. That fear feels awfully real but I have to tell you for a first time mom is highly improbable.

We pulled up in front of the hospital and my husband commandeered an unattended wheel chair and wheeled me into the front entrance. He was going for the information desk and as he was pushing me he just let go to ask where labor and delivery was. I kept rolling, almost to the gift shop. A wonderful nurse took pity on me. 'I know that look' she said and got me in the elevator and up to the right area. A quick stop at the admission desk and I was put in a triage room and told to undress. When the nurse came back to check on me I hadn't gotten undressed yet. Instead of putting me on a monitor she did the dilation check. 6cm and fully effaced. Yippe let's have a baby. My husband went downstairs to move the car and by the time he got back I was in a room and finishing the paperwork. The on call OB came in to introduce himself. It was going to be a crazy night for them. I said nice to meet you but I called ahead for my epidural so if we could get going with that, that would be great. Ummm thanks. Within an hour I had an epidural and I was very happy. I didn't know this but I had a positive Strep B test the week before I had to get fluids on board along with IV antibiotics. The epidural slowed my labor down to a point where I was almost in line for pitocin but it proved to not be necessary. I was happy. I was content. I was resting. The midwife popped her head in a few times to check on me. I was asked if it was ok if she delivered me instead since L&D was getting insane with the full moon and all. I declined. Over 40 with a loss the prior year I wanted a full PhD medical team. No offense. Plus you pay the same regardless. I'll get to billing later but damn many hospitals have flat rates and they are astronomical.

When it came time to push it was just me and a nurse and my husband. I was grateful for that. I didn't require any extra care. As much as I was kind of pissed about being shopped to a midwife vs. an MD I was also blessed and lucky that I was doing so well and was presenting as such low risk that I was having minimal intervention. So this is where my husband's ADHD kicks into overdrive. He's overwhelmed by the moment. He is supposed to be holding one of my legs up as I push and he's distracted and taking phone calls. The nurse is laying into him. I was just concentrating on pushing. I ended up pushing for almost an hour before I was crowning and the doctor and delivery team was brought in. While I was pushing the cadence was pretty simple but it took me a few rounds to figure it out. I pushed twice or three times for the duration of every contraction which the nurse can see on the monitor. Blowing out for a count of ten, getting some air and pushing again. With the epidural you can't tell where you are focusing the effects of your pushing force. I was told to "aim" like I was pooping and concentrate efforts towards that area. That helped a bit. I did feel something tear and some pain at one point even with the epidural veil but other than that I was pretty numb, just scared and tense. So I'm pushing and trying my darndest. My husband is getting yelled at and taking phone calls.

I had the situation where the baby had pooped during labor inside me so a team of delivery nurses came in to grab the baby. It was fine with me actually because I wanted the cleaned up baby vs. the bloody fresh out of the birthing canal version. Once I started crowning, the doctor and a neonatal team of about 4 extra people came in. As the doctor delivered my son he peed on me and the immediately took him over to clean him up. They call the poop meconium BTW which is just super confusing and why can't they say poop. I guess when there is a meconium release they want to clear the mouth and nose right away so during those first breaths the meconium isn't sucked down into the lungs. Makes sense to me but while they had him I was scared. For about 10-20 seconds after he came out he didn't cry and I wasn't looking. After delivering a dead baby not a year earlier I had been scared every minute of this pregnancy. Every kick count every day generated a new set of anxiety and fear. When he finally made noise it was the biggest sense of relief I had ever experienced in my life.
There is a great reality that you don't know bad something is, how much it hurts while you are in it, while are you are doing it. After 9 months of white knuckle daily stress about whether or not this baby was going to live the relief I felt after hearing him cry was like angels singing to me. It was the hand of God gifting me with the most amazing soul to care for. I'm not an overly religious person but I do thank God everyday for the blessings of my

children and for trusting me with their care. What an amazing and pivotal point in your life, the biggest, the best. Rainbows and lollipops.

They handed that little man to me and he looked just perfect. Tired, his eyes were closes, but every inch of his newly born skin was white and perfect and smooth. His head, despite my hour of labor, a perfect shape and not the egg or cone head you hear about sometimes. Perfection. Small. Smaller than I thought. Smaller than the ultrasounds had shown. Tiny. I opened my robe and put him on my chest. Now my parents were in the waiting room the whole time anxiously waiting to see their first grandchild. The doctor took his time stitching me up. And who can forget the delivery of the placenta. Umm yuck. My doctor held it up for me to see. I vaguely remember him telling me by law he had to show me, right before he dumped it in a large home depot paint looking bucket. Extra yuck. He spent more time stitching me up then he did delivering my son. It took about 20 minutes and finally my parents came in to see him. That was a great moment. I found out later that when my husband went to tell them that everything was ok and we had a healthy baby boy he was still green from helping with the pushing and he was ghost white according to my mom and they thought something was wrong. Phew.

The end result. Jacob Aetius. 6 pound 10 ounces. Born April 13th. My sister said since it was the Friday the 13th we should have named him Jason.

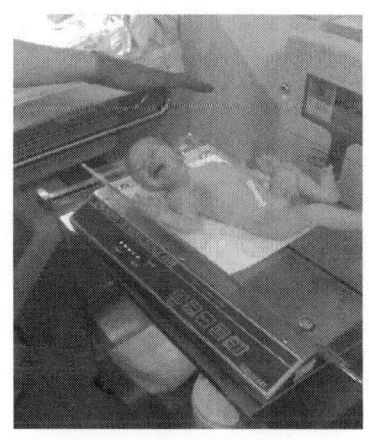

Jacob moments after birth

22. It Just Got Real Round 2. Natural Childbirth And The Ring Of Fire.

The scenario starts at 10pm on a Saturday night. I feel contractions coming on strong and tell my husband it's time to go. We take our son over to my parents house for his first ever sleep over, and head out. I'm packed, we are ready. We get there and the front of the hospital is closed. My husband finds a call box, and has us buzzed in where he grabs me a wheelchair. Up a few floors and we go to the labor and delivery admission desk. I get into triage and have a monitor put on me. Triage was hectic. It was standing room only and the assessment room was full right after I arrived and other women were being looked at down the hall. A nurse comes back about 10 minutes later and says they've been monitoring my monitor read outs and am I sure I'm having contractions because they aren't showing up. Yes I'm sure. It hurts. She stands with me for a few minutes and ask me to let her know when I'm having one. When I said I was having one she said she couldn't see it. About 5 minutes later a midwife comes in and says again they can't see the contractions, so I can go walk around the waiting room area until something happens or I can go home. I opt to go home. I ask why I'm in so much pain if I'm not in labor. No reason given, they were busy and onto the next as soon as I said I would go home. On the way home we thought about picking up our son. We also noticed we needed gas. Neither of those things were taken care of. We got home, my husband had a few beers, not the best idea in hind sight. Then we had sex, not just regular ho hum married people sex, but some crazy ass sweat dripping nc-17 rated movie sex. My husband passed out afterwards. I sat on the floor by the side of the bed and moved between that and stair landing over the next few hours, while I labored and monitored my contractions on my phone. By the time they were consistently a few minutes apart, I woke my husband up and said we have to go, again. This is where the beers didn't help. He was super tired and groggy. He took a shower to try and straighten up. We got in the car and remembered the low fuel situation, so we stopped for gas and a coffee for him. I was not happy in the car at all. While laboring with my son I felt like I could have the baby in the car, during this one I was sure that baby was coming out and I kept my legs closed so tight it wasn't even funny. Screw Suzanne Sommers and the thigh master because I would have blown one of those up I was squeezing my thighs together so hard. We arrive and I don't even want to deal with the wheelchair. We buzz in, hit the elevator and I'm bracing myself against the wall. Back to admission and one of the nurses who was giving me serious attitude while we were there a few hours earlier, asks me if it's for real this time. Don't care and as bitter as I may sound about it I am grateful to have labored at home instead through the middle of night at the hospital. The hospital at 2am is a pretty dismal place. I'd rather be at home with my own bed and TV instead of walking the hallways with my exhausted husband waiting for someone to tell us that I was laboring enough to warrant being admitted and given a hospital bed. Finally another nurse saw the look on my face and took me into triage, which I must have been masked in so much pain that I do not remember, then immediately into a room.

Just as all of the fruit and vegetables at the grocery store are technically 'organic' as they are all carbon based food that is grown not manufactured, all births are 'natural.' I prefer the terms medicated and unmedicated. The newest term is drug free. I can live with that. Well I've had both a drugged and drug free delivery. You can be that person who shows up with your 4 page print out of your birthing demands but you need to talk to God, not the nurses, about that. I had no choice with my little girl. She came too fast and too furious. Thanks Vin Diesel. My first delivery was a stillborn. I had junkie level heavy pain meds and an epidural. My second delivery I had an epidural quickly after arriving at the hospital. This last delivery was completely unmedicated. The anesthesiologist was sitting in the room at one point. Staring at me. Well through his mask I could tell he was thinking 'lady you are screwed.' Proper. To my credit I never swore, I never yelled at my husband, I never screamed, I was never nasty. Just scared. Just petrified. Just completely overwhelmed and encompassed by pain and confusion and anxiety. Several times during the height of the contractions I would utter the phrase "help me, somebody help me." I thought my ass was going to split in two right down the middle. It felt like Thanksgiving dinner and someone tearing the wishbone apart but it was my tailbone and I was being split in two from behind.

During the actual delivery the pain is excruciating. The 30-60 second long contractions did feel like an eternity. I felt completely out of control of my body. She was coming and that was that. My body took over. I wasn't directing anything. I was not steering that ship. After two nurses were finally able to start an IV on me after 6 tries over both arms, one asked me how I felt and I told her I had to push. I was begging for an epidural but you have to have the IV going and like part of a bag of fluids in you before you can get one. They also had to get an IV going to get some antibiotics on board. I had just been told I was 8cm so I don't think anyone was quite prepared. The nurse's answer before hitting the panic button was well if you feel that way then push. The anesthesiologist was still in the room. The kind of crabby nurse, one who shot me a look a few hours previously when I was sent home for what seemed to be a false labor, she is the one who finally got the IV started told the other nurse to call for a midwife and possible delivery. My husband ended up pushed back in the bathroom. I was coherent enough to tell Danielle who was on my right coaching me to get my husband out there and up next to my head. His angle was bad, he would have seen everything as he was in front of me and off to the left and that was not part of the program.

Ring of fire. YES it's real and it burn burn burns. A famous line from the movie Knocked Up "I FEEL EVERYTHING!!!" It feels like someone is trying to blast their way out with a flaming battering ram. Seriously it hurts. So in my blur a few things start happening. The room does go to hell as the nurses start to prepare for delivery. The bottom of the bed has a tray or something that comes out and your feet get rested almost on a platform. Different trays of tools and supplies are wheeled in. As it turns out MY doctor was on call that day, his shift started at 7:00am and as he was making his way into the doctor's lounge someone asked him if he wanted to deliver one of his patients. Me. He was in our room by 7:02, God I love that man I really do. He walked in very casually like "hey how's it going?" That was the last real calm moment we had. I didn't say much, my husband was saved and uttered those famous words "Salzetti is here, it's going to be ok." If you haven't experienced it before, more than likely when you hit the hospital the doctor who actually delivers your baby is usually whoever is on call. For my medical group there were 30+ OBs so everyone did a one day, 24 hour shift delivering at the hospital each month. I didn't have any experience like you see in the movies where you to the hospital and your doctor meets you there, for me it was just luck of the draw who was going to be on call. It was a complete and perfect finish to my baby birthing days. To have my actual doctor who had been on this now 4 year up and down journey with me to be in the delivery room to bring my last baby into this world. Well to catch actually cause she was coming out no matter who was there and she was coming NOW. Dr. Salzetti went out into the hallway to gown up and we were off to the races.

I don't remember who was in the room at this time other than my doctor in front of me, Danielle the nurse off to the right and my husband up above my left shoulder. It all went so fast. I went from saying I had to push, to my doctor coming in, to just pushing, the burn and the pain and just pushing for all I had, not even trying to sync with any contractions, and the true out of body experience that my body had taken over and while I was pushing I really wasn't as I was no longer in control. My shining moment was feeling that I had pooped and announcing to everyone "I just pooped." I pick up dog poop in my backyard everyday, same thing I guess. I never saw it but I saw a nurses hand move onto the area in front of my gapping open maw and quickly away again. Pain and more pain, pushing, burning. Then the halo glows above Dr. Salzetti's head when he says "Two more pushes and you are done." Thank you Jesus. Then OMG SPLOOSH and I don't have any other words for it except that scene in Men In Black when the alien delivers a baby in the backseat of a car and everyone gets covered in slime. I swear I saw fluids shoot out of me and onto the medical staff between my legs, they had plastic shields on their faces and gowns and I got them all with my flying baby juices. Like a cork shooting out of an over shook bottle of champagne, this kid flew out of me, shot out like hellfire. Then it was over and

I was ok. More than ok. The adrenalin of what I just went through, the pendulum swing of this crazy intense pain that I survived BTW, survived with zero side effects, it was just pain and I got through it and it was over and I was pumped, amped, and felt better than I had the last 8 months.

Can I describe having a baby without pain medication? I never planned for it. My bad. I guess I didn't think it was an option that I would be too late. Boo on those nurses for sending me home the night before. Yoda and Buddha, which are kind of the same if you think about it, say that there are no accidents. That sometimes when things happen and its not the way you wanted or planned it's a good thing. Buddha also says chaos is created so that something important that needs to grow can be shielded from your view. You are distracted so you don't interfere. I'm 100% happy with the unmedicated birth of my daughter. It's not what I thought I wanted at all but thank goodness for happy accidents. If I had another, which is sadly out of the realm of possibility at this stage, I would very strongly consider by passing the epidural if labor went fast enough. The allure of the bathtub is intriguing too, but I feel like I've had a full range of experience and though it was the hardest the unmedicated birth of my daughter soup to nuts was by far the best. I had some experience under my belt at that point so I kind of knew what to expect and it was the quickest by about a factor of a hundred. My induced labor for our stillborn baby took about 14 hours from getting checked in and the first dose of pitocin to actual delivery. My second delivery I was in the hospital a little under 8 hours before he arrived. My last was under an hour in the hospital before she shot out like hell fire. Love that kid. She was always crazy, even before she was born. The most active by far and the most trouble.

Truly as with all of my deliveries it's a bit of a blur but the time my doctor came in until the end it didn't last more than 15 minutes all together. Every other minute of that very short time was consumed with mind bending, body splitting in half, pain, but even then that level of intense pain lasted less than ½ an hour. I speculated later that one of the reasons they probably sent me home a few hours earlier is because my labor wasn't showing up on the monitor well as it felt like it was all in my back and the bottom part of my butt. For someone who was not prepared in the least for an unmedicated birth, I did my best. I didn't read, didn't take any classes and really didn't even pay attention to my yoga instructor who also taught the Bradley method whenever she would talk about breathing because in my arrogance I figured it wouldn't apply to me. That having an epidural was my choice and I wasn't opting or hoping for a 'natural' birth, so of course that is what I got. Au natural was supposed to be for those antioxidant taking millennial girls in my yoga class who are doing their downward dogs the day before their due dates. Not old, jaded, sarcastic, kind of sour and not so warm and fuzzy all of the time, me. The nurse who was coaching me did an amazing job. She was calm and directed. Ok she kept saying "great job," "you are doing great" and 'breathe" which was like ehhh I didn't need that but that's me. Told you the breathing would come into play, a lot. A younger more sarcastic me would have told her to STFU. I didn't want to hear it from my husband but I tolerated it from her. What I needed I got at some point which was my doctor telling me where the end was. 2 more pushes and the baby will be out he said. Excellent. A end point to focus on. I can't tell you how much that one piece of information helped. Tremendous help. Like struggling during a workout at the gym and looking up to see 2 more minutes of cardio until you are done. You can make it. You can push for those 2 minutes. Hell you can even accelerate and take it up a notch if necessary and you can instantly get into a "let's kick a little ass" mood when you can see a clear end.

The delivery room was chaos. Despite everyone's best intentions the fear you feel is real and its from so many different angles. Fear for the baby is paramount. The few seconds after my son was born and before he cried was the slowest most emotionally painful and fear filled 30 seconds of my entire life. For real. I was a the top of a 100 story roller coaster peering over the front car waiting for the drop. Fear for you. That comes and goes. The pain and lack of sleep and food amp that mother up about 1000 fold. With my son I hadn't eaten in almost 36 hours before I had him and only slept about 4 in the same time period. With my daughter I hadn't slept in about 24 hours and hadn't eaten in about

12 but I also had had sex and labored mostly at home. I also had the additional anxiety of dropping my son off at my parents house for his first overnight. That was tough too. The separation of having to leave him with them. I became scared for those three, my parents in having to watch him without me or my husband available to assist and for my son being left alone for the first time with someone other than us. Scary. I was afraid for my husband. He's an absolute rock but I know hospitals and doctors and all of that isn't his favorite thing in the world. He forges on during all of these events but I do worry being a loving and devoted wife that he is afraid or not being well taken care of. With my daughter it all went so fast and our doctor was there, as opposed to the random doctor on rotation, so my husband was good to go.

There is so much you don't know and can never know about the workings of the hospital, the hierarchy of the nurses and the doctors and all of their interplay and protocols. Part of being brave is being afraid but still having to let go. It doesn't hold truer than in this case. You have to put the trust in the hands of the people who do this all day every day. Still they can be pretty terrible about explaining things. Just because it's automatic to them and they see it all of the time doesn't mean you understand the process in the slightest. From the monitors to the IV's to the sequences to the timing its all a totally new experience for you and actually if I was in charge I would make sure all nurses and doctors kind of calmly explain how things go. I wish during my epidurals that someone had explained to me how the process goes instead of just doing it. Maybe that is a bad thing. Maybe explaining things generates even more fear and anxiety. Knowing what is coming can make you be tense right? Well I think not knowing is even worse. There were so many things I wasn't scared about being in the hospital the last time. I had some of the routine down. I know that you get an IV and that it lasts for a while. That actually went out the door this last time because they couldn't get it started after several attempts it finally ended up in my hand but because I had natural delivery as they call it was shortly removed. When I had an epidural with my son the IV stayed in for almost a full 2 days and that felt worse than the loads of stitches in my lady parts. I've talked to moms who've had all types of different experiences with the two extremes being a scheduled c-section and an at home birth with midwives. The difference between scheduling the event and having it over lickety split, and having an inflatable pool in your living room.

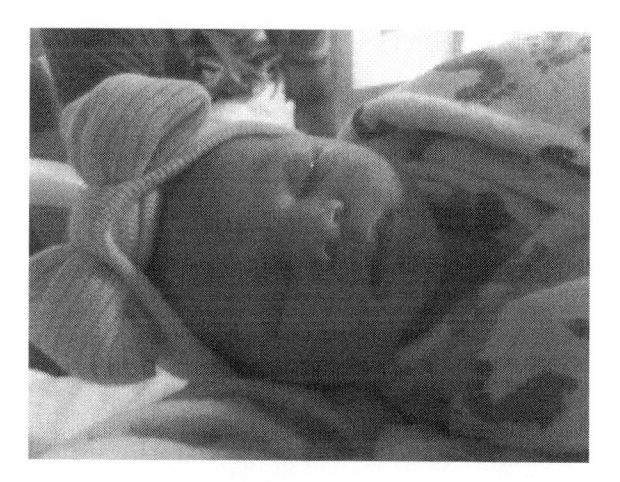

Elizabeth Grace

Elizabeth Grace Ramirez, born after college football on Saturday and before NFL football on Sunday, cause I'm a dope ass wife about my husband's football. Shot out like a cannon. September 7th at 7:17am weighing 7 lbs. 7.7 ounces. She's a living breathing Super Lotto jackpot.

23. L&D Game FAQs Player Game Walk Thru.

So as best as I can recall here is your step by step guide. It's not even close to being complete but it's my best attempt based on my 3 hospital experiences.

This all starts with getting knocked up. But seriously lets fast forward.

1) A decision to go to the hospital must be made. This seems trivial and a given but I found it hard to find that threshold. In fact this can be the hardest part and time management is of the essence. In some cases the decision is made for you if you have a scheduled induction or c-section. If your water breaks, seems like a good sign you should head out soon. In my case I had to make my own judgment calls. Yikes. I felt very ill equipped to do so. With my son I was having contractions for almost 12 hours before we decided to go. My husband actually decided for us. He saw me get doubled over with a contraction in the kitchen and pointed out that I was a tough person and for something to kick my ass it was probably real and serious. He was right. I think we are really poor at judging this very important tipping point in the entire process. There is a lot of fear and not knowing with not having gone through it before. The what if I'm wrong and have to turn back around coupled with 'is this it' real or false labor and for me the real factor was I did not under any circumstance want to spend a day or two in the hospital in labor. The doctor and nurse given parameter is 511. Contractions 5 minutes apart lasting 1 minute consistently for 1 hour. Yeah I never ever experienced this BTW. The closest I got was deciding to go to the hospital again after being sent home when having my daughter. I downloaded a contraction tracker app for my phone and had 30-45 second long contractions every 3-4 minutes. Great resource and I highly recommend it, track your contractions on your phone so you can really see a chart of the progress. By the time I got to the hospital we were so far down the road already. I had her less than an hour later. With my son I was glad I waited as long as I did. I also never had my water break at home. I found that when you are beyond the point where you can have a comfortable continuous conversation and are a little distressed for a bit on a regular basis, that's a decent tipping point. Most women panic and that involves them being in the hospital for way too long before that baby comes. My amazing yoga teacher handed out little words of wisdom at the end of each class. One was to really try and listen to your body and the longer you spend in the hospital before delivery the more likely you are to have a c-section or induction. That makes sense actually. If you are having a long drawn out labor you will probably need or want intervention. It's a tough decision. Would you rather be in a hospital bed for 2 days laboring surrounded by medical professionals or at home having contractions and being a little uncomfortable. I'd rather be at home without question however if you are scared or in trouble go to the hospital at the first sign. It's not something to mess with. Always remember you are not in control of this and even with a ton of experience, which really no one other than those nut job Dugger women have with their 20 babies, things can go sideways in a minute. And even with all of their birthing babies experience they still have issues, you don't really know if the baby is in trouble without a heartbeat monitor etc. They will send you home if you aren't ready. I feel good about both of my decisions though maybe cut it a little too close with my 2nd. With my son I was in the hospital about 6-7 hours before he arrived. With my daughter less than 1 hour. I can live with that.

I really feel that this is one of the most important decisions that impacts everything. Once you are in the hospital and checked in with IV's going you are not leaving until you have a baby. That means no food, no comforts of home, and everything that entails. Enjoy those ice chips and the 6 channels available on the micro TV with the broken remote on the uncomfortable bed with your husband looking pretty lost and wanting to be anywhere but there for the next day or two. Did I mention as soon as you are in there is no food? None. No eating. However do yourself a favor and don't gorge on the way over, it's not worth it. I saw some baby show on TLC once where the woman went into labor and had the taxi stop for bagels and smoothies before she went to the hospital. Pass on that. I love food more than most and haven't skipped many meals in my lifetime but I didn't miss it for a second while I was in labor. And in case you don't know why you aren't supposed to eat it is a precaution if things go south, which you cannot predict, and you need to have a c-section or have emergency surgery and they go to put you under and have to place a tube down your throat to deliver oxygen. If you've filled your belly you could throw it all up and it could settle in your lungs and stop your breathing and really hurt you and hinder the process of putting you under where time is of the upmost urgency so just don't do it. You always hear that you aren't supposed to eat after 10pm or midnight the day before you go in for surgery, same thing sweetheart. I had a fruit bowl and a Caesar salad at 11pm after my son was born. Yum. Best food ever. Worth the wait. I don't remember eating at all after my daughter was born. Not the entire day. I'm sure my husband brought me a yogurt parfait, yum by the way and one of the best options from the cafeteria, but I don't remember doing anything other than trying to talk the staff into letting me out asap and nursing my baby.

2) The check in. We arrived at the hospital safely, which my husband did best all 3 times by just pulling out front. Put that on your list of things to figure out before you have to go to the hospital is where you are going to get out and how you are going to get to labor and delivery (L&D.) Our hospital had a large front area, like valet parking without the valets. My husband was able to leave the car out front while we went and got checked in. Sometimes you can even find an empty wheelchair. It in the middle of the night however there is no one to help you, and we had to use a call box and be buzzed into the L&D wing elevator section. It's not like there is a doorman or anyone waiting out front to meet you and help you out. I actually walked up the very last time. Cut down on all of that wheelchair stuff. You don't need it. You and your husband have to be with it enough to figure out how to get to the labor and delivery front desk in some of the most chaotic moments of your life. Trust me your cool calm husband will be in panic mode as one of his main jobs is getting you to the hospital. Good luck. I had assistance the first time by a nurse who took pity on us. Since my doctor was already in their system and this was our assigned hospital etc. getting checked in wasn't a problem. My medical files were already on board and once they pulled me up I was escorted back to the L&D triage room. This is one of those times where you need to be an adult and do adult things before hand spending time and energy figuring out what your insurance covers, where your in network hospital is, etc. Some women do a complete pre-admin. I recall briefly filling out a form that went on file, but I was well versed with what my choices were. They will need you to confirm your ID and your insurance information. You have to keep in mind this is a business and they need to get your billing trail going asap. There are tissues and trays and all kinds of fun charges to send to billing so they need your info so it goes smooth. How else are you going to get charged $50 for the few newborn diapers you used. Thank goodness we didn't have to make any alternative decisions. I can't imagine having to call to see if a different hospital took my insurance. The worst case scenarios are out there. I have a friend who didn't do her fact checking before hand. She was married but forgot to put herself and her new baby to be on her husbands insurance. She went where she wanted to have her baby, what? The closest hospital. No biggie right? Wrong. Her bill was over $20,000 that she is still paying off 3 years later. All because of a lack of spending an hour or so to try and figure it out. I would fight very hard to save that kind of money. Very hard. I was fighting with the insurance company over $100 worth of lab work. After 3 pregnancies in 4 years and dozens of tests and office visits and 3 deliveries I felt like I left about $120 on the table in costs I didn't look at closely enough when they were billed. I went over my delivery bills very carefully. There was some nonsense on them for services I didn't use. One bill had a $2000 charge for nursery services. My son spent approximately 4 hours in the nursery over 2 days for his real first bath, his circumcision, and while I slept for a few hours at the nurses' insistence. With my daughter she was at the nursery for less than an hour for her first real bath and that was it. I don't know if you have choices everywhere but our hospital gave you a rolling bassinet with supplies underneath and my daughter never left my side. I thought that's what everyone was moving towards but I still had the exact same nursery charge on my detailed bill. When I called both the insurance and the hospital it was a standard flat fee and the total billing for a baby is practically the same using boiler plates for the few different types like a c-section vs. vaginal etc. You are going to be a parent so get your act together and figure out your insurance before you drop that kid. Also keep track of your expenses on a spreadsheet, as all of our out of pocket medical can be tax deductible along with the miles traveled to and from your doctor appointments.

3) Triage or as I like to call it the first of many times someone's hand will be all up in your Kool-Aid that day. You get undressed in the bathroom and into a very attractive, soft, and figure flattering hospital gown. In one of my cases I couldn't get my own shoes off. My husband was downstairs moving the car. The nurse had to help me undress because my contractions were already on top of me. You put your clothes in a plastic bag with handles and then lay on a table. A monitor is attached to your belly. The nurse reads the strip and then lifts up your hospital gown to determine how dilated you are. Just an aside I trust the medical professionals but with my 2nd I had a midwife read the strip, I was having contractions but all of my labor was in the back so the strip didn't look as consistent as it should and L&D was crazy busy so I got 'streeted' as they say in the medical lingo. I was lucky to get back in time before my baby came. After it's determined whether you are getting admitted or not, which is a nurse looking at a monitor and read out and trying to see how dilated you are, you are either instructed to get dressed and go home or walked over to a delivery room.

4) **Getting the Hook up.** A few different things happen at once during this next time period. A nurse is assigned to you to get you set up. You get into a bed. A monitor is attached to your belly. They start setting up an area for you and your things. An IV is started. With an epidural my IV stayed in the ENTIRE time I was in the hospital and the IV site hurt worse than my lady parts for about 5 days. If you've tested positive for strep B a bag of IV antibiotics is hung along with the saline. The admission paperwork is completed. The doctor on call pays you a visit to introduce themselves. With my son this is where I had requested an epidural so the anesthesiologist came around to administer that. You need to have a bag of fluids on board before they will start the

epidural in most cases. I've read in some hospitals they have a threshold point where they won't do it if you have progressed so far in your labor. Our hospital's only policy was a bag of fluids on board. With my daughter I didn't get 1/8th of a bag on board before she started crowning.

This is also a time where we settled in to our room. My husband parked the car and went to get a cup of coffee. You have to find the TV remote, the bed control and nurse's station call button then make all of your calls and send your texts. Try to remember anything you forgot to pack and bunker down for the duration. After the epidural with my son I actually kind of drifted in and out of sleep for the next few hours. As this day truly is all about you and your needs, more so than your wedding day and enjoy it because it will never be all about you again, well at least for the next 18 years, set that aside for a second and make sure your husband is **FED**. Seriously. Even if you aren't that wife that takes care of your husband just make sure the guy has a drink and a sandwich. You are going to need him later. You need him awake, calm (good luck) and able to make good decisions for you in case something goes wrong later. I would instruct the nurses, who are your allies and can act on your behalf, to make sure he knew where to get food and the cafeteria hours etc. At 2am its impossible to get anything done in the hospital except getting woken up to have meds, but there is some food to be had if you ask right. Usually turkey and cheese sandwiches and yogurts that are kept at the nurses station. Finally, you can hear the monitor next to you, if it's been turned down you can ask for it to be turned up. It's tracking your contractions and the baby's heartbeat. This is where the staff can see if the baby is recovering well after the contractions. This is important. If they baby is NOT recovering well after contractions that can be the tipping point to a c-section.

5) More about "The Juice." I feel this needs some more detail. I had 2 epidurals and wanted a third for delivery 3. You tell the nurse and doctor you want an epidural. Then you wait. There is usually always someone on call, however you don't know how busy they are. You could have a serious wait so don't wait until you are so consumed by devil pain that you can't see straight because if you wait until you can't take it anymore the chances you will get any type of immediate service is absolutely zero. Again be a grown up. Use your brain. I know it's hard but there really isn't a scenario where you dying and want big time pain relief and the anesthesiologist is totally available to service you right now. Duh. With my son it was about 30-45 minutes. With my daughter I actually did luck out and he had just finished giving an epidural down the hall and he was in the room ready to work on me but I was too far along to get one. Bugger. So here is the protocol. Are you ready. First you get a catheter. Yes because you are numb and can't walk to the bathroom or control your bladder so a catheter is inserted. So not fun btw. Yuck. Actually a little discomfort but not real pain. They grease up the end of a small clear plastic tube and the nurse inserts it. Then the juicy juice man (or woman) comes in. When vacationing one year down in Turks & Caicos there was a lovely gentleman who used to walk up and down the beaches a few times away. You know him. Yes it was the weed dude. Same kind of thing here. He is the guy in this joint who has the good stuff. You are asked to sit up and pull your back taught by rounding it towards the doc, arched so your arms and shoulders are forward and your back is curled. The first time my husband held my hands. The second he was out getting coffee and I had the nurse hold my hands. Yes have someone hold your hands. Its scary. Large giant needles are going into your spine. It sucks. It hurts. Not like labor pains hurts but it's scary and you are tense and it's sharp and frightening. You need someone here to help you. To keep you calm. I was contracting through my 2nd one and it was no fun to also have the fear of trying to stay still on top of the big giant horse needle in the spine fear. So the location is sterilized with the orange benadine stuff. Then I believe a plastic like sheet is laid on the surface. Then shots of lidocaine to numb the area. That is no fun. Lidocaine in general, anywhere, is not a treat. It's a sharp little needle that stings. Like a nasty wasp sting but it goes away much quicker. Ok here is where it gets weird and during contractions tricky. The 2nd needle goes in, which is hallow then the cathedor is inserted that will feed the pain medicine into your spine. OMG so much fun. So weird feeling. For one of mine it went in kind of at an angle so coming out it was oh not so fun. You are then basically confined to the bed from this point on. I know there are walking epidurals but I didn't have one. In my case I fell asleep after both, probably passed out from the stress. The pain relief is pretty instant with a total numbing in less than 15 minutes. I will say that with both I was not in toe curling screaming bloody murder pain. I was in pain, I was uncomfortable but it wasn't even close to being at that unbearable threshold. I strongly advocate that as the optimum time to juice up. Not when the demons are on you and you've lost your mind in an abyss of pain. The relief was very very welcome and I was able to relax with the birth of my son up until the time I had to push. Your legs are numb so you aren't going anywhere and that numbness lasts after delivery and for a bit after the epidural is removed. So now you have a whole bunch of things connected to you. An IV with fluids and/or IV antibiotics. A baby monitor on your belly. A cathedor in your pee pee attached to a bag secured under the table. And a cathedor in your back hooked around up onto the IV pole. Yeah you aren't going anywhere until that baby comes out. Period. So do anything mobile you want to do before hand.

6) **The Great Wait**. Hurry up so we can wait. I am blessed to the heavens. I did feel a little stir crazy waiting the few hours to have my son. Made up for by the absolute chaos and immediacy of shooting my daughter out a few short years later like wildfire. The TV sucks. Your husband is anxious. There are only so many texts and email and phone calls you can make. What did we do before our smart phones for real. I can't imagine. So hurry up and wait. You will be checked on by nurses and midwives and maybe even a doctor or two. Every few hours they will put their hands in your ever widening vagina and tell you how far along they think you are and evaluate your progress. Your husband will be insanely bored during this time. He can only text and call so many people. Make sure he has an ESPN app or something to occupy his mind and his time or he will be talking to you driving you nuts. I didn't have that but I've heard. As much as I wanted my husband there to be at the birth of his child, really I felt like I could have done it all by myself. Its kind of miserable for them. Think about it if the shoe was on the other foot. Imagine sitting in a hospital room where everyone is addressing your husband

instead of you and he is in excruciating pain or worse in jeopardy and there isn't anything you can do about it. Plus you are bored out of your skull. On top of it hospital food sucks but mine was too scared of leaving the property in case something happened to go get himself some decent food. That's where a good hearted visitor would come in handy. If you are a 3rd wheel visiting while someone is in labor, bring food for the hubby. Something really really good. He needs it. And coffee or a red bull por favor. Gracias.

7) The main event. Here we go. At some point someone will tell you that you are now 10 centimeters and fully dilated and it's time to push. Or not depending on the circumstances. With an epidural I didn't feel much so it was a bit of a surprise when a nurse came in and checked me and said it was time to start pushing. I pushed for about 45 minutes before my son was crowning and a doctor came in to finish the delivery. Up until that point it was just me and the nurse and my husband. She held one leg while he held the other. Up and at a 90 degree angle. You can hear them and the nurse can see the contractions on the monitor. With the start of the contraction deep breath in then hold for 10, then a quick breath and hold for 10 then another quick and hold for 10. That should take you through the contraction. You aren't deep breathing during the contraction, you are holding your breath and pushing. You are Tom Cruise in any Mission Impossible movie holding your breath an abnormal amount of time. With an epidural its hard to figure out where to push. I mentally focused on a spot between my cha cha and my butt. Like I was pooping. However with all of that numbed drug haze going on I still felt something rip while I was pushing. Not my parts but maybe an abdominal muscle (?? as If I had any left) but I felt a sharp pain right between my right hip and belly button. With that baby I did not poop. I didn't have to. I hadn't really eaten anything and I made sure I went before we left for the hospital after I took my very very long shower and shaved. With my 2nd not only did I poop I announced "I pooped" to the room. It's kind of expected. In theory you are using the same muscles, motion, etc. It is quickly removed BTW by professionals who see it every day. No biggie. Far nastier things are going to shoot out of your crotch in a few so don't sweat it.

Please have enough sense to make sure your husband is where you want him. At some point during the chaos of my 2nd delivery my husband ended up looking at me from the bathroom, in front of me off to the left. He was trying to get out of everyone's way as the room when to chaos and ended up backed into the bathroom. As soon as I saw him I put a nurse in charge of making sure he came up above my shoulders for the actual delivery. My first full delivery was a relaxing experience. 45 minutes of pushing then the doctor came in for the final little bit. I also had a neonatal team in the room. The little guy had pooped in the womb and if they inhale any of that after delivery its not good. So after just me and the nurse and my husband all of a sudden there were 8 people in the room. It's a floor show with the Holland Tunnel you call your vagina up front and center for everyone to see. Final push and out he came. They kind of pulled him out sideways to get his shoulders out. And he peed all over me. He also didn't cry right away. Now that was frightening. The worst part of all of it. The doctor handed him off immediately to the neonatal team for clean up and to make sure he didn't get any poop down his throat, etc. Eye drops. Then they weigh him and do a reflex test. Then I got a baby with a knitted cap, swaddled in a hospital baby blanket back. Heaven. I opened up my shirt after a few minutes to nurse. That skin on skin contact immediately after delivery is highly recommended, and during your entire hospital stay of course and even with your husband too. Slap that little on his hairy chest. They love it.

So while this is going on, my husband is snapping a few photos. I have a great one of my son on the scale after his reflex test, he looks like he's doing karate and an amazing shot of him in my arms right after they handed him to me. Also while this is happening a few minor details are being cleaned up. The delivery of your placenta then stitches.

8) Clean Up, Aisle 5. While you are blissfully distracted here comes your placenta. My first doctor held it up so I could see it.

Uuumm yuck. A bloody squid covered in bloody snot is what it looked like to me. Then he chucked it in a white medical waste bucket and settled in to do my stitches. He was chatting away and he really took his time. I wasn't even paying attention, fixated on my beautiful son, who had already been cleaned up by the neonatal team, who then finished their protocols and left. A side note on OBs, they often have the gift of gab and I haven't met one yet who won't strike up a conversation when they are elbow deep inside of you mostly as a distraction technique. The stitches that time felt like they took an eternity but I didn't actually feel a thing because I still had the epidural. I do remember being very anxious because I couldn't have my parents come in until they were done and I wanted them to see the baby and they had been waiting their whole lives for a grandchild in addition to the whole day at the hospital in the waiting room. The second set of stitches were not as pleasant. My daughter came into this world with a furious sploosh which sprayed everyone in the immediate area which I could see on their gowns and masks. With no pain relief on board I was then administered several lidocaine shots to numb the area so my "front to back this time" tear could be stitched up. I felt every stitch and then some. The area was super sensitive as I had just passed a whole human being through it not a few moments before. It was swollen. It was on fire. And now it was stuck with 4 needles and being stitched. I got some super fast down and dirty stitches that time and it was everything in my power not to clamp my legs together to stop him from doing them. I know I was wincing and moving. In direct contrast to the grace and elegance and almost plastic surgeon type approach to my stitches the first time around, my doctor went as fast as he possibly could. I was begging for an epidural just for the stitches. I was turned down. I also didn't get a cleaned up baby this time. I got a wiped down baby but she was nasty dirty still. In her first pictures I can see blood and other goodies right above her left ear in her hairline. Her other side was highlighted by a kind of squished nose and the top of her right ear was a little screwed up. My husband got a similar round of pictures. Baby on the scale and baby in my arms. I held her first, she got swaddled right after delivery so I held her first then they sucked out her nose and mouth, weighed her and did the eye drops then gave her back. With my first I stayed in the same room for quite a while. Maybe because of the epidural. That ended up being the room I stayed in until the next morning. With my second I got moved into a recovery room within the hour. Since I didn't have an epidural the 2nd time and hadn't been able to get IV antibiotics on board before she came, the IV port was removed (such a blessing) and I got moved into a room in a totally separate wing.

Do keep in mind during all of this that the nurses see the worst of you too. Be prepared. I tried to shave before going to the hospital to have my son. Looked like Amish LSD quilting patchwork. Not good. The professionals really don't care and don't judge, well not that we know of. Let's say they judge your behavior not your body. Bring CHOCOLATES, Dove Chocolates are best. Individually wrapped with little cute notes. Give them out to the nurses. All of the nurses who come in your room. It works. Quality of care rises. If you have an epidural the nurse has to help you to the bathroom the first time. They are checking you out to make sure you aren't losing too much blood and help you assemble your post pregnancy pussy pacifying pie. Disposable mesh panties, plus a rack and crack ice pack, plus tucks pads plus numbing foam. Heaven. You can assemble good replicas at home. This is where the chocolates are helpful so instead of remembering you as the patient with the giant blood clot you are the nice lady who had a cup of chocolates on her tray. Better. After my last baby I wanted out of the hospital ASAP. I was told in order to do so I had to be vigilant about reporting any clots. Oh boy I had one the size of a small Chihuahua that I saved in a pan in the bathroom for the nurse and doctor to look at. Disgusting Jell-O mold of left over baby producing fluids and membranes. I also never took a shower in the hospital. It creeped me out. I waited until I got home.

9) Visitors. Your call. I've had both good and bad experiences. I know couples who tell EVERYONE that they are at the hospital and EVERYONE shows up at some point or another. During labor. No thanks. Afterwards. No thanks either. After my son was born I had two sets of visitors I wish I hadn't had. One was my step daughter and her mother. Loved seeing my girl but could have lived without her mom being there. At the time we were all getting along great. A few years, a multitude of court battles, and having her turn very nasty towards us and towards our children as well it's hard to look back and see pictures of her holding my newborn son. Before my sister or anyone else other than my parents held him. Loved seeing my step daughter but I don't have any pics of just her, it's all with her mother and her mother holding my son and as it turns out later that was by her mother's design. The son she now won't acknowledge and the son that proved to her that any chance of getting back with my husband was gone and it sent her over the deep end. The other visitor we had was my estranged father in law and his girlfriend. After not speaking with us for a year they showed up unknown to me (thanks honey) and caught me as I was coming out of the bathroom with a blood soaked gown trying to call for the nurse to bring me a new gown and more supplies and they were staring at my blood stained sheets. No thanks. It was about 2 in the afternoon and I had just survived the visit from my husband's ex wife and now I had a whole bunch of drunken nonsense. Yes they smelled like they had been drinking and smoking. No I wouldn't let them hold my baby. They hadn't talked to me in a year. My father in law walked out of our lives the day we lost a baby the prior year. He hadn't called, he never told me he was sorry or supported me during that pregnancy, that loss or the current pregnancy. And here he was. He actually didn't want to see me and really didn't want to see the baby. My husband smartly took him away from me and tried to direct them both into going down the cafeteria for a cup of coffee. His father went, the girlfriend did not and spent the next 45 minutes giving me her two cents on babies and her daughters new age hippie philosophies on food, diapers, everything. The gift basket they were generous to bring, she had assembled with 2 huge jars of coconut oil and a bundle of all natural biodegradable diapers. She educated me on her philosophies which she picked up from her Millennial children about not using baby lotions, different feeding techniques, etc. I didn't pay attention. I just wanted to get out of my bloody gown and off the bloody sheets and I wanted her to take herself out of my hospital room so I could rest and be with my baby. Their visit ended up extending into the evening where they invited my husband out to grab a bite to eat.

Well since my father in law hadn't talked to my husband in over a year they had some catching up to do and he kept him out for over 3 hours. I was by myself, in the hospital with a brand new baby while my husband was out with his father and I was scared and exhausted and mostly furious. Don't let your having a baby be an excuse for someone's family reunion. Looking back I was very disappointed that I allowed some estranged family members to put a damper on the most special day of my life. With my daughter I had learned my lesson. I had one set of family friends visit at the same time as my parents visited with my son. I got to introduce my son to his sister, then our friends showed up with flowers and for a very sweet photo op. About an hour later everyone left and I was able to rest. That is the way to do it. You are in charge and it's your velvet rope into your event. Don't let anyone else dictate or bully you into visits.

10) Congratulations. Your baby will go to sleep almost immediately after delivery and stay pretty sleepy most of the rest of the time. It's been a long and hard journey for them. Stick them on your bare chest until you have to go to the bathroom, then you will figure out on the fly how to gently place a sleeping baby into a bassinet and get ready to deal with the rest of your hospital stay which is a bunch of nonsense really. Lots of administrative protocol, etc. You fill out quite a few forms like the application for a social security card and birth certificate. Do yourself a favor and take your time on those, you have nothing but time to get these done right. Total pain in the ass to make corrections later. Our hospital had a contract with a company that sends photographers around for your baby photos. Ehh. Buy a set. We did. They are terribly overpriced but it's a memento of your journey. My son's are amazing. My daughter's not so much. $50 for a couple of prints which is ridiculous since you just get print, no digital copies, those are extra. Even the mall Santa gives you a digital photo in their $35 package. The two photographers we had seemed like maybe college students as the college was less than a mile from the hospital. Very nice and experienced at set ups and positioning babies but I felt like I had cooler pics from my phone plus I could text mine out vs. waiting for paper prints. They also put your info in their database to call and email you relentlessly over the next year for your FREE or discounted sitting with their affordable, $300-$1000, set of prints. It's genius really. Who is going to turn down buying gorgeous prints of their new baby after a 'free' professional photoshoot. It's not like the Splash Mountain at Disneyland where you feel ok to pass on the sloppy eyes closed photo of you plummeting down the waterfall.

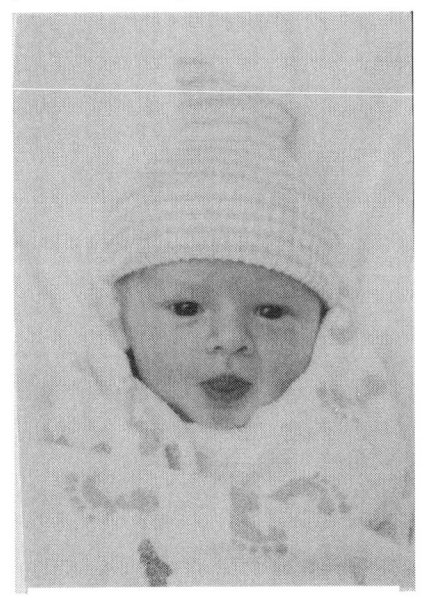

Jacob's hospital photo

I had to get the DTAP vaccine right after I had my son and I believe I had a booster about a month before I had my daughter. Get your shots. Seriously. Do NOT mess around with this. Have your family get them too if the are going to be handling the baby. Jenny McCarthy was wrong when she came out publically against vaccines. Well intentioned, but misinformed. As a former Playboy employee I will say that YES Jenny is certainly one of the most witty, smart Playmates but no virologist or PhD of infectious disease. Don't be swayed or influenced by the millennial holistic philosophy to not vaccinate. Get your shots.

You have something to eat. You can actually find some decent choices on the hospital menu and send you husband to the cafeteria for salads and yogurt and fruit. I stuck to salads, fruit, yogurt parfaits and bran muffins. I drank a decent amount of juice and a ton of water. All I cared about was getting out. I nursed my babies. The first time I had a bunch of nurses instructing me on how to hold him to feed him. Football vs. cradle, ugggh. Last baby I actually had lactation specialist watch me nurse and check and adjust the latch the baby had. Now that was helpful. You end up making a lot of small talk with a lot of different shifts of nurses. As previously mentioned I kept a bowl of Dove Chocolates on my tray and offered them up to the nurses. They are doing their job. The majority of them I found really love babies or they wouldn't be working labor and delivery recovery. They are a wealth of information and will show you how to nurse, change a diaper, swaddle, and all types of other handy tips and tricks. Listen and learn. Let them teach you. You don't have to use their techniques but it's good to have extra things up your sleeve when you are tired and out of your mind in a few days. I let my son go to the nursery for a few hours the first night. I did not do that with my 2nd. I only let her out of my sight to have a real bath and a few tests so I could take her home. The nurses are in charge of following up on you and your basic health, blood pressure, temperature which can spike if you have an epidural, etc. They will monitor your output, pad usage, and your general condition. I was a little taken aback having a nurse help me put on and change a pad and monitoring the output. I passed a huge clot on baby #2 and had to save it to show the nurse. Yuck. It was the size of a small watermelon, really nasty gross, and definitely horror movie special effects quality. With baby one I went through tons of gowns and sheets and just bled everywhere and didn't have a good handle on it and I was a bloody mess for 2 days. I asked where to put my bloody sheets and gowns and was instructed to put them in a corner and housekeeping would come get them. I seriously went through a dozen gowns and about the same on the sheets. With my daughter it was much more manageable and I was better and dealing with it and very proactive about changing out my pads et. al every 2-3 hours regardless whereas the first time I was kind of waiting until I filled everything up but most times the fluids come out with tsunami like mass and velocity. I was also peeing all over myself with the first delivery, I don't know if it was the epidural or what. I think it might have been. Anyway you interact all of the time with the nurses. Lots of taking your temperature and blood pressure and monitoring your oxygen level and monitoring your post delivery bleeding as well as tracking your feeding of the baby and the baby's diaper usage and output. They will wake you up to give you an Advil and a Colace and to check on the baby if you have them with you. Lots of poop and pee. Welcome to life as a parent. Its kind of what it's all about. I used the same hospital each time so I'm not sure how other hospitals handle their protocols. I had to have a certain level of stability and an exam from the OB on call to be cleared to be released. My son during our 2 day stay had blood tests and a circumcision, which if you are going to do it, do it in the hospital at day 1, seriously. It's less trauma for everyone to do it right away and not wait a week. That is one decision you need to have talked about or hopefully have made before you go into the hospital. I was hesitant but don't regret it for a second. I felt like a monster discussing cutting part of my newborn son's penis off, but then again it is standard, there are arguments both pro and con, however if you are going to do it, do it right away. I was told he didn't even cry but I wasn't there. Like the belly button, it's a piece of skin that falls off a few days later all Jeff Goldblum "The Fly" like. Then he had to be cleared by the pediatrician on call to be scheduled for release. My daughter was a little more complicated because I had tested positive for strep B but didn't get an IV antibiotics on board she needed blood tests as well as a follow up with my regular pediatrician 24 hours after release just to make sure she was ok and didn't catch any of my nasty coochie germs. Trust me you'd rather pack up and take the baby to the doctor the next day then spend another night in the hospital. That I don't regret for a second. It's no fun going to the doctor on day 2 with a butt full of stitches and a newborn BUT it's infinitely better than another night in the hospital. When they tell you you are officially cleared to be released it can take a few hours for all of the details to come together. You have paperwork to sign and go over. My hospital gave you a kit for how to care for your baby, a prescription for pain killers and a bunch of forms to get generate and get copies of the baby's social security number, birth certificate, which costs money to get in my county from the recorders office, etc. Basic instructions about how to not kill your baby and basic care and a chart to keep track of feedings and diapers. Good solid info. You have to show on the on call nurse that you put the baby in the car seat properly. Since most infant seats have the detachable carrier that was easy for us. My husband when he brought the car around front remembered to bring the carrier up to our room. Finally on your way out take everything. You technically paid for it as part of your hospital charge. Take the diapers and the wipes, any pacifiers they give you and the thermometer. Take all of the pads, cream, witch hazel pads, everything for you too. You need a total kit to take care of your lady parts and trust me your insurance has been charged a small fortune for all of it. If I told you that you were probably charged around $5 per diaper and $10 per pad, would that compel you to take them and use them? Well then load up that bag and hit the road.

11) We are Going Home. Oh that first car ride is rough even if you've done it before. It's stressful and scary and anxiety riddled. With my son we had him in the seat properly but we hadn't adjusted the base of the seat to the correct angle so he was at a bad angle driving home, much more far forward than he should have been so his neck seemed to be strained. Not ideal. I installed the car seat in our driveway which is on an incline so I didn't get the base adjustment made to have it be level when he was in it. Corrected it immediately after we got home. I had one of those neck support pillows but it didn't really fit right so we opted not to use it. Had it down by the time we were taking our daughter home but it's still a tough ride. With my son I rode in the back. With my daughter in the front. With my son I was jumping out of my skin with every bump and bad driver. With my daughter I wanted her to sleep and I took it easy. With my son I came home to a house destroyed by our dogs. Very Lord of The Flies as no one had checked on them for over a day, and while they had food and water they pooped and peed everywhere out of protest for being left alone, so I had that mess to immediately deal with. I was wound so tight and totally stressed out from the drive and the bad angle on the car seat and needed a shower and didn't want to deal with anything. I never showered in the hospital so one of the first things I did both times was take a good shower. Wash off all of that blood and hospital smell. The dogs always knew I had been in the hospital and kind of stayed clear. I think after my shower I put on some cozy clothes, yoga pants and a cotton cami and a nursing bra then settled in to feeding the baby. Then a big deep breath. You can finally relax a little. You want warm, you want cotton, you want an ice pack in your pants. As a shower gift one of my friends gifted me with things more for me and one item was an ice pack you could fit in your underwear. I used a travel pillow to sit on, it was kind of like one of those old folks butt pillows. Brilliant.

12) Here starts the BLUR. I don't remember many details from those first weeks with either baby. I remember the 2nd being easier to juggle than the first but with so much more anxiety because my first was then a toddler. It was like Jackass at my house and I was so petrified every time I needed to lay down or nurse that he was going to escape into the street or set the house on fire or try to climb on top of the refrigerator. I remember managing the bloody aftermath a million times easier due to a few factors including not having an epidural, not being in the hospital as long, having an easier and much much quicker delivery and being overly prepared. I was military like preparing for a major offensive and all I got was a little skirmish. Don't get me wrong small blessings. I loved it. I had everything from a pack of underwear I could totally throw away to pads and Depends and numbing foam and witch hazel and ice packs and even a travel pillow / butt donut. Didn't really need it but was glad to have it. I remember my nipples hurting. With my first the anxiety of being a new parent set in immediately and culminated with an extreme amount of stress over my lack of breast milk on day one and breast feeding in general and having a ridiculously difficult of a time getting going. Every annoying factoid that anytime you tell you doctor about a problem you are having or physical symptom their first response is "that's perfectly normal." Ugggh. My issues with breastfeeding weren't a problem with my anatomy or the delivery system as much as it was about my lack of knowledge. The hold, I got too many suggestions at the hospital and I got confused so I kept changing holds. For all of the hold advice I got with my son, I got no latch advice which is all I got with my daughter. The latch really is the key and how to correct it when it's going south on you. The hold will work it's self out and may be different with different kids. You will figure out the position that works best for the both of you. With my first I supplemented right away and it totally effected my output. With my second I exclusively breast fed from the get go and was slower in introducing solid foods too. I can shoot milk across the room this time around. There still is pain though. When I say it's a blur, I have overall impressions and notes from one of the newest busiest weeks of my life. So much to take in and process it's insane. The specifics of that first week in particular are truly gone. I remember going to the gym about a week after my first one. Not so much with the second. I just took it easy. That is my best advice for that first week. Don't plan a thing. If you have family and friends who want to visit, great!! They have to bring food and be able to give you a break, even if it's watching the baby sleep for a few minutes while you go to the bathroom, take a shower or at most a quick nap. Did I mention they must bring food and they must be self sufficient? This isn't about having a visit with you or you waiting on anyone, making a meal for your in laws or scrubbing down your bathroom. Your job for that week is to just take it easy. Be good to your body. It's experienced more trauma than most people endure during a car accident. Your brain is cooked. Your body is exhausted. Just focus on you and your baby. Feeding and sleeping both of you. Being warm and snuggly. I wanted nothing more than to be in bed surrounded by my dogs under a warm blanket. This is your week, you will never get it back so just be good to you. It's one of the few last times you'll be able to do so for a very very very long time.

24. My Best Delivery Room Advice.

Leave the multiple collated copies of your birth plan at home. It ain't happening. If you do get an experience along the lines of what you had hoped for then you are blessed and it's a miracle and be grateful. The problem comes when things do not go as you want them to. I have a close friend who spent months training and planning for a hypnobirth. This is a technique where you use hypnotism as your pain relief. She ended up going a week over her due date and had to be induced. It left such a bad feeling for her even months after her beautiful daughter was born. She was pissed, disillusioned, disappointed. Don't set up one of the most miraculous days of your life with the potential to walk away disappointed or to leave a bad feeling that lingers because your expectations are too tight or too rigid. You can't really control what is going to happen. If your baby is in distress you are having a C-section. Period. No doula or hospital is going to risk your life and the life of the baby because you want to stick with your breathing techniques or you had your heart set on a water birth. I don't mean to sound mean but really let it go. It's in God's hands for real. You can control if you want to TRY having an un-medicated birth vs. an epidural. That's the latitude you have. By all means try. But if you hit transition and end up getting one drop of that sweet sweet relief you will be kicking your own ass for not having done it sooner and suffering as long as you did.

Get a good general array of knowledge. I watched videos, and read books and did yoga. I wish I had investigated natural birth techniques a little more. I also wish I had been more educated on c-sections and by the grace of God I didn't need that info but if I had I wished I would have done more research.

Are you sitting down because here comes the real advice. The price of admission. The reason you bought this book.
LISTEN TO THE NURSES. Hello they deliver babies everyday. So much so that's its marginally unremarkable to them depending on their moods. Yeah it can be clinical but it's the means to an end. The bottom line is that you have your baby. The method makes for a good tale that it's fun to tell birth stories for the first

year or so but afterwards ehhhh no one is interested and truthfully the only ones who give two hoots are your mom and any friends you have that are expecting. I look at the 36 hours I spent in the hospital having my daughter as a necessary vehicle to get to the end game which was my beautiful healthy child that was delivered in an environment that made me feel safe, made me feel like if anything went wrong they could take care of her properly and that's about it. I don't shower there, I don't poop there. I'm in. I'm out. Get me home so I can be with my baby.

The nurses know when to push. The nurses know how to breathe. They know when you are in trouble. They know when your baby is in trouble. They can teach you how to nurse, swaddle and change your baby. They know everything. They've seen everything. Be good to them. Do not swear at them. They are not your maids. Don't be a pig. I know it's hard. With my son I was in the hospital for almost 2 days and I went through a dozen gowns and sheets etc. Do what they tell you to do with your trash and dirty linens. They are there to help you but don't be a jerk. They've seen it all. They are your comfort during delivery. For my son a sweet nurse Jackie was holding my left leg and timing my pushes and breathing. During my daughter's delivery it was heaven sent Danielle who was my birthing coach and saved my life by helping me focus and get my breathing on track. The doctors are like the figure heads. They bip in and out but the nurses are in the trenches with you. They do the work with you. Be kind. Bring them treats. Maybe Starbucks gift cards?

Regarding your husband and his position in the delivery room remember some things cannot be unseen. Seriously. Your lady parts while pregnant are really for exam by authorized personnel only. If you don't have an MD or an RN stay away from the birthing zone. Do you really want your husband to see you open up and expel a head out of your cootch, along with the blood and alien pouch placenta? No you don't. Once you get some sleep in a few months you'll want him to want to have sex with you again so keep him up above your shoulders. It's for the best.

25. General Comments For The Aftermath.

As I'm re-reading my yoga instructors newsletter about all of these issues surrounding delivery I'm baffled. Was I blessed? Maybe. The big message in the natural birthing community that I kept hearing over and over again was to avoid medical intervention at all costs. That the longer you are at the hospital the higher your changes of being induced or having some type of intervention. I guess this is a dual edged sword though isn't it. If you are high risk, like I was, or nervous or a even a first time mom maybe you do need to be in the hospital for monitoring and it's almost impossible for you to tell how far along you are in the labor process. Laboring at home as much as possible is a great concept. It makes sense that if you are in the hospital for 2 days laboring they are going to induce you if for no other reason than to reduce your suffering and undue stress on the baby as well as limiting the liability of the hospital. I was in labor and delivery 3 times and at no point did I ever feel pressured towards a medical procedure. The only thing that I didn't really sign off on per say was after my epidural during my son's delivery I kind of nodded off and my labor slowed down. Which according to the first medical team that saw me was a good thing because they needed to get fluids and IV antibiotics on board. After a few hours however then I was told my labor had slowed down too much and I needed pitocin. I never actually got the pitocin as my labor moved along without any issues but I saw how quick they were to prescribe that and it went on my son's medical birth record that I had it even though it was prescribed but never administered. It's part of a demographic that was submitted to the state. 42 years old, vaginal birth, pitocin assisted.

It's their job to get your baby out. So yes the longer you are in the hospital the more they are going to try and get your baby out of you. I guess that leads to feelings of loss of control. Umm Duh?!? Call me crazy but I never ever imagined that really any part of my delivery was in my control, well as soon as I hit the hospital doors. I knew if I wanted to eat first, which god love your body with all of my deliveries I had no appetite for hours even a full day before as minor labor pains had started. I wanted to take a shower and poop in my own toilet with no one around instead of during my delivery. All of that needed to be done at home. If I wanted to walk or have sex, yup at home. Cuddle with my husband, ehh do it at home. The hospital is about lying down, texting, dealing with the medical staff, and that's about it pre-delivery and monitoring contractions, filling out paperwork, chit chatting with nurses, watching your very bored and fish out of water husband try to occupy his time, these types of things. After delivery its about feeding your baby and having all of their medical items taken care of, bath, blood draw, circumcision, etc. and managing to eat what the hospital and the cafeteria have to offer. I've also seen women post delivery complain about lack of pain relief as well as having a painful and lengthy labor. No offense ladies but that's kind of what you signed up for. I'm shocked that this shocks or annoys anyone. Seriously. Now I understand I'm lucky, everything that happened to me was very straight forward and without a lot of crisis with the minor exception of how fast my daughter came out. I never cursed or screamed at my husband, not once. It's like losing control and blaming it on drinking too much, I always found a way to be in control of my own actions and this was no exception. I was in more pain than I had ever experienced in my life and scared to death but I didn't feel the need to get primal about it. If you are in that much distress that you want to get all Exorcist in the delivery room than for the love of God opt for the epidural, seriously. Do you really want your husband to have the memory of you calling him a cock sucker who did this to you? No, you want the magical unicorn riding a rainbow image of your child's miraculous birth.

Punched in the pussy along with your period on crack.
You will be bleeding for a while. At least a week if not longer. After my son was born I bled off and on for 4 weeks straight along with a bladder I couldn't control. My daughter was kind of the opposite. I was in panty liners for the bleeding by the end of the first week. Word on the street would be because I had an drug free or what some call a natural delivery on my last the recovery was sped up. I do agree with that for some and that my body was already a little adjusted for the rest. I had a few giant blood clots in the hospital, uggh they looked like nasty Jell-O molds. Or

something out of one of those shows on SyFy where you make monster movie effects. Disgusting. The bleeding however was really light. Awesome.

Put your pride aside and stock up on supplies ahead of time. Grab your CVS coupons and go to town. After the baby comes is not the time. You will be tired. You will be stressed. You will be out of your mind. Buy a pack of depends. Buy a 6 pack of granny panties you can throw away later. Buy a small box of Colace. Buy a bunch of tucks pads. Buy some poise pads and panty liners. Buy enough for a month. Do you really want to send your husband to the store for pads? Didn't think so, so stock up before baby. Thank me later. Get your 2 foot long CVS receipt and start buying all of your supplies about a month in advance. And take ALL of the supplies they will let you take from the hospital. Everything. You paid for it so take it, pads, numbing foam, shake and crack ice pads that go in your panties, diapers, wipes, all of it. Make your panty sandwiches. Disposable panty or granny panty. Plus a rack and crack ice pack pad from the hospital. Layer on some tuck pads like lunch meat and add some numbing foam on top like whipped cream. The Colace is so you can poop, take one if you haven't the day after you get home from the hospital and keep them close for the next few days especially if you decide to fill your vicodin prescription from the hospital. That will back you up too. My friend bought me a peas ice pack from the CVS that I put in my panties. Ice is your friend. You are swollen and sore and stitched up and the ice does wonders. Don't be proud either. Your husband just watched you shoot out a baby. If you want to sit on an icepack and a hemorrhoid pillow for 2 weeks do it.

Hitting your due date. I hit mine. With my son I actually had 3. One based on the calculation from the first day of my last period. One based on the extensive ultrasounds I had and where the baby was tracking. The third was from a phone app I had downloaded. There was only one discussion ever about having a c-section and it was at my 8 month perinatal appointment where my son was estimated to be over 8 lbs at the point. He wasn't BTW. Keep in mind some "measurements" are really extrapolations given other measurements which are only as accurate as the eyesight and mouse clicks of your ultrasound technician. They make points on the screens when they measure leg bones et al then other measurements are calculated off of those and like all things human interpretation is flawed. One of the reasons I was so so thanking the lord above that I never had to make the impossible decision of being given a grim result on a genetic test of my child. What do you do? I felt I was not that person who could raise a severely handicapped child and I would have opted to end the pregnancy. But how can you be sure? How many tests and experts do you need to see before you can be absolutely certain? And all before legal termination deadlines. It's crazy.

Going into labor. Now since I didn't go beyond any due dates so I can't tell you what that process is like. I've heard its almost daily appointments during which you are begging your doctor to either induce you or not and they are trying to figure out what is best. One of the philosophies preached by the holistic faction is that without intervention the body does what it is supposed to do. Word up on that. My body went into labor and my hunger was shut off and the process began and I made a point of taking a poop before I left the house. Especially with my last baby my body took over 100%. I really felt like I hadn't control over what was happening. Instead of pushing her out I felt like she shot out. I couldn't stop it. With my son I had an epidural as soon as I arrived so I was reliant on the monitors and medical staff to tell me when to push and it was kind of a long process about an hour or so. Yes if you can withstand the pain and God willing it goes quickly having an unmedicated birth is the way to go. Having the medical staff there to catch and support is the optimum. Not everyone is that lucky. It's a crap shoot and you absolutely don't know what you are in for until it's on top of you. It's not like you can feel labor starting and start weighing your options. Well this labor feels like it's going to be smooth and problem free so I'll go to a birthing center instead is the hospital and opt for a tub instead of a hospital bed. I ended up in that bed 3 times. I have friend's who have never experienced labor with any of their kids due to scheduled c-sections. This is a growing trend in the wealthier set just like birthing centers are for millennials.

The hospital sucks. I would have much rather preferred the tub and to not be surrounded by monitors and medical staff and that hospital smell and feel but I'm also a realist and I know if something went wrong that is where I had to be. Not in a tub trying to desperately figure out if I needed to go to the hospital and trusting that the person directing my birth knew when and how to get me there if I needed it or more importantly the baby needed it. Better safe than sorry? Hell yes. Every time. Does the hospital suck?? Beyond. I hated it but that's the sacrifice I had to make. It was a short part of the experience and I did everything to get out ASAP. Maybe that is what comes with the 'maturity' of being an 'older' or late in life mom. You are rational. You are pragmatic. You are logical. The years of being swayed by trends and peer pressure are long behind you, well kind of, maybe, hopefully, at least enough to make a good decision for you about where to have your baby. At our age I don't think you really have a choice. Would I rather have been sipping on tea with relaxing music and dimmed lights soaking in a tub. Oh you better believe it. Instead I got all mine in at home. Before going to the hospital with my son I took a marathon shower and got organized. That made me feel like a million bucks. With my daughter I went to the hospital then was sent home because my labor wasn't trackable on the monitor. So I went home, had hot sex with my husband, and after he passed out labored in my bedroom for the next few hours. During contractions I would kneel next to the bed and when they got stronger I would hold onto our stair landing for support. I enjoyed being at home and got mines at home. Don't expect any love, privacy, or good vibes at the hospital. Sure the nurses are usually super nice. Sure you get the added security of knowing you are in the safest place for your baby. But it stinks and it's uncomfortable and you cannot absolutely cannot rest. All I did was countdown until I could leave. But having the baby glosses over all of that. means to an end. All that matters is the end. Well don't forget before you go home there will be pictures. Maybe lots of them. Hair and make up before delivery, kind of useless, my sweat and exertion melted off any drapings of civilization I tried to apply before giving birth. Afterwards is probably the best time but good luck, I was so wrapped up in nursing and holding my baby and not wanting to put them down for a second that I wasn't going to excuse myself to do hair and make up for the close up after delivery shots. They aren't my finest look but they are pure and they are genuine. They are some standard shots you might want to be prepared for. You with baby. With that horrible hospital gown on. Daddy with baby. Other siblings with baby. Hospital beds are nasty backdrops so find something more suitable.

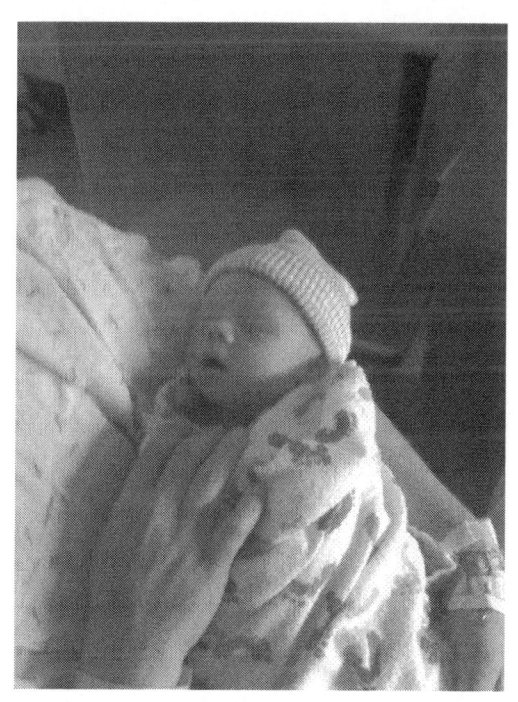

Holding Jacob for the first time

The first picture of me holding my son, Jacob, is one of my favorite pictures ever. Taken by a very green husband right after delivery. As mentioned the hospital gear, like the red hazmat garbage can, always looks horrible in the background as well as those terrible gowns but what can you do. I love this photo. That's my son. He's perfect. They had to clean him up before they gave him to me and he's already asleep after hitting the baby trifecta of pooing, peeing and crying. Nap time.

The next picture is me and my little girl. Is that the same gown from the other picture 2 years later? The little hat with the bow on top handmade by hospital volunteers. OMG. After I texted out a photo of my little girl I got a response back telling me to take that God awful ugly hat off of her head. You know I guess it's actually a picture of me after one of the most physically intense few hours of my life. To myself I look absolutely awful but the moment is so important. It's all about my hands in both photos. My hands on my baby. That's what you should focus on. I have different angles of the baby right after this photo was taken but this captures a moment that I'll never forget. I was practically Kourtney Kardashian wanting to reach down and pull that baby out of me even though it wasn't 100% cleaned up. With my son I didn't want blood and yuck on him, with her I got her eye drops and a quick wipe but she didn't get a real bath until later and she still had blood and stuff on her hairline. I didn't care. I wanted her in my arms. She's red and puffy and squished and her nose is off to one side and one of her ears is all melted but at that moment she was out and she was mine. She was an anxious to get to me as I was to hold her.

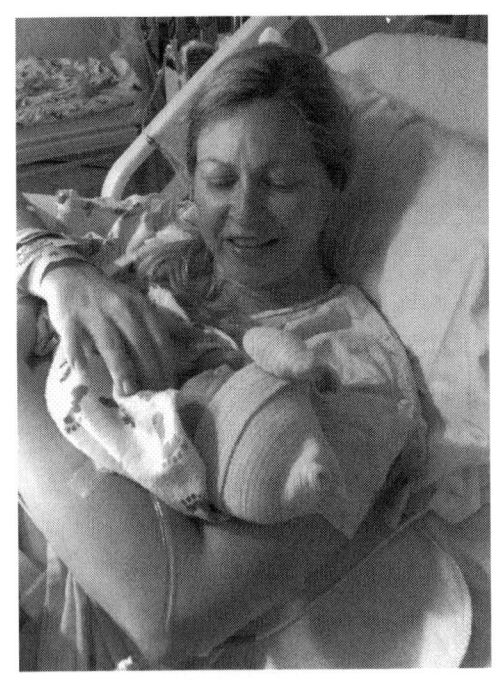

Me and my baby girl

26. Things I Was Surprised By.

The list is large. After the birth of my son my first big surprise was how difficult and painful breastfeeding is. How much my nipples hurt and how much they were damaged. Bloody, cracked, bleeding, painful, OMG over the top 20 on a 10 scale pain. I heard rumblings here and there that some women have issues, but my God, it hurts. On a good day you feel nothing, on a bad day it's like Deadpool is motor boating you and playing ping pong with your nipples.

I was also shocked that totally losing bladder control for about 2 weeks was a side effect of either the epidural or the delivery. Not sure which but no one told me that I'd be peeing on myself without any ability to control the flow. In case you didn't know regular pads don't hold that type of liquid very well. It's too watery. I ended up calling my doctor on this one, and I was a very low maintenance patient during that pregnancy and that was my very first phone call into the doctor for over two years. None during my pregnancy or pre-pregnancy. His solution was tough to hear. That if the situation didn't correct it's self or I wasn't able to gain some control through Kegel exercises that I would have to have bladder surgery.

I was surprised that no matter how hard I worked out I wasn't going to really drop any weight for 2 months. Minimum. There was also no real boomerang effect and all of my dieting and exercising during those first 8 weeks were nice and all and got a good routine set up but really didn't from my view contribute to my weight loss.

I was shocked that when I went in for delivery I was informed by the staff at the hospital that I had tested positive for strep B, I didn't even remember having a test for it. That I had to have IV antibiotics before delivery. During the delivery of my little girl, which happened too fast and furiously to get any meds on board before she shot out, I was again informed that I had tested positive and needed antibiotics. So you can imagine my panic when I realized that not only wasn't I able to get an IV on board so I could get fluids in preparation for an epidural, totally missed the window on that, but I also didn't get the bag with the antibiotics. That scared me to death what I was going to transmit to my wee one. She was fine though, thank goodness. No issues.

I was surprised that the epidural slowed the labor down and that I was able to rest. While filling out the birth certificate I was also shocked about a mistake that was made related to this. Whether or not you had an epidural ends up being part of the birth record, the data collected by the state for statistical purposes. At some point during the delivery I was prescribed pitocin to speed up the delivery after the epidural et. al had slowed it down. However I never received it as my body kicked in and delivery went forward without any further issues. Because it was on my medical record it became part of my son's birth record. I tried to speak with the nurse on duty in recovery to have this fixed and the person who worked for the hospital (I think it was a social worker?) who helped complete the birth certificate information didn't really seem interested in helping me correct this mistake. Said it didn't matter. It mattered to me though. One thing no one really understood, especially those who worked at the hospital and were a little jaded to the daily business of delivering babies and bringing life into the world was that I was doing a lot more than having a baby. I was moving statistics around. I was gaining street credit for not only myself but all women out there over a certain age. And if my birth record said I had pitocin and I didn't and I was probably one of less than 5% of the women who delivered that year who were over 42 that skewed the data significantly. I had and have a responsibility to all women over 40 to make their lives less stressful and make the statistics better for all of us.

I was surprised by a lot of things during my first loss. I was surprised that my child was small and had a cord issue. I was surprised no one had really sat down and talked to me about it, that it was there or what it meant. It was mentioned but not discussed. I didn't know what the potential issues were. I read about talked to the doctor about it but still was totally caught off guard by all of it and didn't understand it until after she was already gone. It didn't cause the loss directly but that was one scenario where I saw God's hands at work on me. I was surprised how after the initial devastation of the loss I felt ok about everything. I was at peace within a few months, getting pregnant again right away helped tremendously, but I felt like ok this is what happened, it wasn't my fault, I have to move on. Almost absolved, that nothing I did contributed to her demise though some issues in my past tormented me a little and gave me pause for thought, I felt secure that nothing I did ultimately led to her death. It was a fluke and coming from a scientific family helped me process that better. I know many women who are emotionally sidelined and depleted by 6 and 8 week miscarriages. It haunts them for years. I am not haunted. Once I reconciled that hey this was not in my hands and I did absolutely nothing to contribute to this loss, I was and am really ok with it. My husband probably took it harder than I did. He got very upset when the hospital sent us an invitation to a candlelight vigil it was hosting for families who had lost babies. We were sent home with a condolence card and a card with her footprints. That was hard enough.

My surprise for baby number 3 were not nearly as earth shattering. I was pleasantly and joyfully surprised that the new Sequenom assay, MaterniT21, being able to identify issues via a 10 week blood test on me was available and accurate. Accurate enough that me at 45 with a loss in my recent pass could bypass having an amniocentesis. Unreal. I was also surprised that there was going to be no way that I couldn't find out the gender of my future baby. With all of the testing and medical care comes a ton of information. Information you can't unsee or ignore. In this case my husband was told gender at week 11 when the results of the MaterniT21 came in. That 'secret' lasted less than a week as I overheard him telling someone on the phone.

Nobody told me that:

> While in the hospital the nurses would be so pushy about nursing. Lord help you if you chose not to nurse and go straight to formula.

> That as you are nursing those first few days your uterus contracts to the point where it hurts as much as labor contractions. Well beyond a bad period cramp type of pain. My friend had to use a heating bad on her stomach before and during nursing to help with the pain

> That nursing sometimes feels like someone putting knives through your nipples while your baby is feeding. After my son was born nursing was far more painful than labor.

> My neighbor shared with me that no one told her that with a c section you look down that first time and it's drinking Frankenstein festival. Cut from end to end.

> That the hospital can be absolutely awful. I kind of thought of it as neutral before I had my son. It's disgusting and after you've had a baby and you are bleeding and peeing everywhere and you feel disgusting and the hospital is disgusting you just can't wait to leave.

> Everyone has that 3rd trimester panic with a toddler in the house already as to how am I going to do this? I had a little boy who was climbing on counters and shooting out the dog door how was I going to nurse and keep him from hurting himself at the same time?

> Stitches can hurt more than delivery. Stitches without anesthesia after a baby just passed through your lady parts is a mind blowing intense pain that must be akin to getting shot by a gun and has to be the work of the devil.

> You worry that your husband / partner will be turned off by your pussy which has pushed out a human being and been stitched up and it will never be the same again and he won't want to have sex with you ever again. So sorry not the case. Men really don't really care about these things. Pussy is like pizza. Even bad pizza is still good.

> You worry that your husband will be turned off by your boobs as they start to shrink after nursing. Again they don't care that much, or I should say that maybe I'm lucky and mine didn't. Wear a push up bra.

> That while you are worrying about your weight and your boobs and your stretched out vagina all your husband really cares about is you and you as his wife and as a parent to his child. It's so cliché but if the love is there before baby, and you survive that sleep deprivation of the first year without biting each other's head off, the love grows exponentially. I sound silly and sentimental but it's true, the respect and love we have for each other is so immense after having our children. Makes me tear up. Tito get me a tissue. Jermaine stop teasing.

> That people you don't think of as being part of your inner circle are going to be so generous and sweet and so happy for you it will warm your heart and strengthen your faith in humanity.

> That people who are part of your immediate family will not celebrate for you and it will piss you off and hurt your feelings. I'm still waiting for my children's only uncles to acknowledge their existence.

> That some family will use the birth of a child to mend old wounds and make new bonds.

> That other family members will be so jealous of your good fortune they will pull some stupid stunt to put the focus back on them instead of your new baby.

> That you are amazing and your tolerance for pain is far beyond what you ever thought it could be. That when you put your mind to it and focus on the end results you can overcoming going through procedures and situations that you never thought you could handle.

I never intended on having an umedicated birth. Ever. Ever ever. But I did it. I didn't have a choice. Sometimes when you don't get what you want it's the luckiest thing that could happen. If I had another baby, and I think about it a lot that I would love one more but we've pushed our luck so far already I would do my best to have an unmedicated birth. I would even love to try a birthing tub. It's all life changing, and as much as you hear that you aren't the same person as you were before you had children, it's 100% true. There's no going back now and you wouldn't want to anyway.

IV: After Baby: And Now the Fun Begins

27. Sunday Bloody Funbag Funday

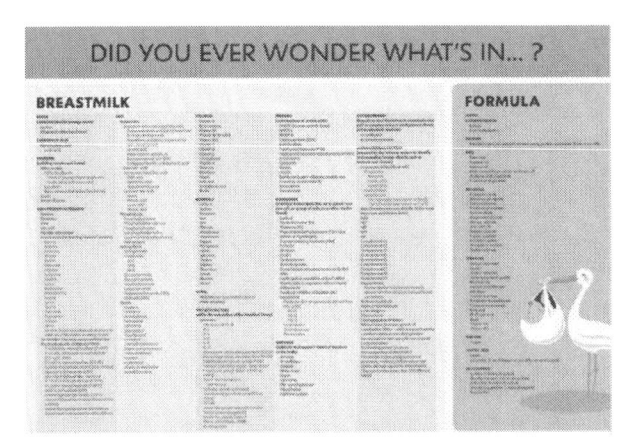

You get the picture, breastmilk GOOD

Regarding breastfeeding. You can read all about it, get a lactation coach but it's still something you have to do and experience to figure out. One singular characteristic on the above chart should strike you above anything else. Formula and the nutrients it contains isn't even in the same ballpark as breast milk. This doesn't even take into consideration the bonding and healthy hormonal benefits for you that nursing provides, that's just a straight up ingredients list.

I powered through because it was important to me and my husband. As the oldest of the new moms in our social circle I was the only one who put the time in to nurse. With my first I panicked on day one when my milk wasn't in so we immediately started supplementing with formula. I was cool with that. It allowed my husband to feed him so not only would I get a break he would get that bonding experience. I had a hell of time getting going. It took over a month for my son and I to sync up and get a groove going. I had blisters and scabs. I was in constant toe curling pain and the worst were the times my son threw up my blood because my nipples were oozing. It took 2 months for my nipples to have any resemblance to a body part again vs. the skin of a desert lizard. They hurt, they bled, they were a disaster. I also got a bout of mastitis. Woke up around 3am shaking uncontrollably. Took 15 minutes to get up the strength to wake my husband up to take the baby and feed him. I was a wreck for a day. But I powered through.

By the time the next baby came around I learned a few lessons. Not to panic and to relax about it. I was obsessively concerned about my son's weight and how much milk he was getting. With the last baby I exclusively breastfed and found my supply to be more than abundant and she is more than well fed.
Every once in a while I do a check to see if my supply is still flowing. I'll give my nipples a squeeze. Most times and I haven't learned my lesson yet I end up squirting my face and into my hair. Yup still work. There is this underlying doubt about breastfeeding. Unless you see the milk actually flowing into their mouths I have never stopped feeling scared that maybe it isn't enough. That I'm not producing enough. That they aren't getting enough. With the bottle you know exactly what they are getting, you see it, there are lines so you know down to the millimeter ho much they've eaten. With your boobs you have to have faith, trust, which is very difficult when you are so tired. Doubt always creeps in when you are exhausted and scattered. Having more than one child allows a lot of your doubts and fears to fall by the wayside because you are so busy and constantly pulled in different directions you have no choice but to believe that what you are providing is enough but with that first one I had a quasi-panic constantly about providing adequate amounts of milk for my precious beautiful baby.

With baby number two I fed in public, I fed anywhere and everywhere. Always with discretion, no one especially old dudes and young boys need or want to see you breastfeeding. Think looking at that lady walking around naked at the gym. Yeah no. one of my best experiences was feeding my daughter at the San Diego Zoo. This was right before our very evolved and family friendly community was smart enough to put a dedicated nursing station in the park. BTW it's absolutely disgusting. It's a walled in area about 6 feet wide by 10 feet long. Right next to a first aid office and serves as the main diaper changing station with a bench and a shower curtain for feeding and everyone leaves their poopie diapers there so it smells disgusting and makes you want to vomit while you are trying to nurse. It's also downwind from one of the main animal enclosures so while I give the zoo major props for putting in this designated area, it's gross. Anyway before that I found a remote and isolated bench one visit to the zoo. I placed the stroller in front of my as camouflage and always used some light weight blankets to shield my body and the baby. I'm sitting on this bench. The sun is shining and reflecting off of the pond that I'm overlooking and I'm surrounded by all types of different wild birds including flamingos and ducks. Amazing.

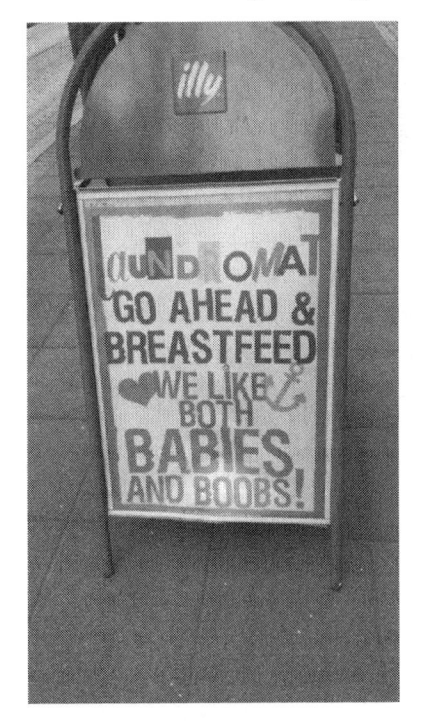

Original Source Unknown but we love it

I also did my fair share of feeding in the car. Bring a pillow for that one to support your arm and the baby properly. The occasions we were out watching a football game or some other function I would just shoot out to the car to nurse. Works wonders if the baby gets fussy and gives you are good excuse for a break. There is something very tranquil about sitting in the car in silence feeding baby. Do remember you car isn't as private as you think and try and cover up. As pro breastfeeding as I am I don't want to see your big old blue vein boobs out on display. It's not that hard to get a light blanket and cover up. It's like being in the locker room at the gym. God love those ladies who walk around naked, but I don't want to see it, it makes me way too uncomfortable.

Nursing has been a gift. For me. For them. My family doesn't even notice it anymore. I took some selfies of my nursing. They are kind of out there. You can see most of my boob. Is it too much? I don't know. A family friend send she wouldn't bring her preteen boy over because she didn't want him to stare at my boob. I was pretty free about nursing in front of folks, with a blanket of course but sometimes things get exposed. I agreed with her. If her kid was going to get weird about it, It would be best to keep it from him. A friend of mine came over while I was nursing, now I was a bit more unrestricted around women vs. men. I have nursed in front of my dad, but with a lot of blankets and covers and of course my husband but that's it. Men get grossed out but what I came to realize it's the women that stare. This woman came over one day and I started nursing my daughter under a thin cotton blanket and she kept staring and asked how I got her to latch on so quickly. She hadn't had luck nursing and I found out later due to having had very pronounced enhancements done to her chest. She didn't try but that is her choice. I don't care what you do, this was my choice and I was doing it I was just surprised by the reactions of women, really kind of gawking at my nursing. That one caught me off guard, I expected more of a female solidarity in the form of ignoring it like you would in the locker room at a gym, you look but you don't "look.'

How to beat a boss and breastfeed at the same time
One of the interesting aspects of nursing is figuring out how to be productive with that time. I would usually sit in my recliner or lie on my bed for hours at a time. Yes you are already being super duper productive as a matter a fact as about a productive as a woman can be feeding your child. However, your mind can

wander and I used my time nursing to work on items on my phone either games or communication and to play Xbox. I remember distinctly getting some good video game time in. I beat a lot of bosses and got quite a few levels unlocked. That's the rub about nursing, it's really really hard to multitask. Multitasking while nursing is an art form. With my son I was so concerned about production and if he was getting enough that I sat, I sat in the same area in the same position and it took me a few months to get a good position down so I felt good about his latch and how much he was taking in. I wanted to be still and tranquil and focused. With my daughter I just slapped her onto my boob and have no problem walking around and doing small tasks. I do wish I had gotten one of those wraps / carriers where I could put her in and give her a boob and call it a day while I go hands free. A boobie blue tooth if you will. I would have so used that. I am at the point now where at 25 lbs. I have had to become much more limited with what I can do while she is nursing. You really do have to sit. You can walk around a little to do small tasks but it's hard to type or do anything that requires a lot of precision or dexterity. Based on my extensive experience things like curling your hair and doing your make up are out. Thankfully she nurses for shorter times now or while we are in bed so I don't have all 25 lbs. pulling on my war torn nipples. She is ornery though, and sometimes will start to screw around, joke around, wildly shake her head from side to side while she is clamped on. It hurts now. I'm done. My poor boobs are already looking like sand in socks even though the production is still top notch.

I'm so thrilled that celebrities are advocating nursing. I'm beside myself that the hospitals do too. It's awesome but it is hard and it is a choice. It would be like if the re-useable holistic diaper advocates were down your throat at every turn. I tried those. Ehh. Got them for free from a friend who had invested quite a bit in the system. They weren't for me. So I moved on. That's how a lot of people feel about nursing. But the time does get kind of lost while you are doing it. It ties up your day, it ties you into a location. So to see celebrities post pictures nursing on set, in a dressing room, while getting hair and make up done, it's fantastic. I'm savoring every minute with my last one because it is the end. Such an easy way now to comfort and sooth my little girl, to get her to sleep, to get her back to sleep when she wakes up.

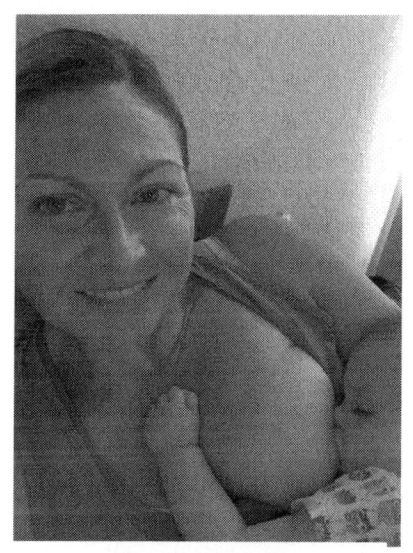

Nursing Elizabeth

The advantage of being the later in life (LIL) mom is that you have the mental and emotional maturity to really squeeze every drop out of these experiences. These treasures that you didn't even know where there. You will know when it's time to stop. I did feel I stopped too early with my son but the signs were there. He was fidgety, didn't stay on the boob long, and became quickly distracted and disinterested. My little girl on the other hand will ask me for boobs, she says please and practically rips my shirt off. Seriously she is sweet about it, she says please and pats my chest and then sometimes lays her head on me. It's precious. Aside from being a free and practical way to nourish your child, and trust me when the cost of cans of formula stack up real quick, it's a cliché bonding experience. One you'll never want to give up because there is such a closeness to feeding your child and the warmth they feel from you and you from them. It's comfort. So man up and do your best. So what if your boobs go south afterwards. Make a cast of them while you are pregnant then if you are older you should be set enough to get them adjusted later on.

Boobs vs. Pacifiers

Never used one. Tried a few times but always found a boob to be more effective. Neither one of my kids did the pacifier thing. My son puts anything and everything in his mouth but never used a pacifier. I know mom's who have that plug in their kid's mouths well into the toddler years. I personally sucked my thumb as did my cousin. We both did so well into our pre-teens and my cousin used to have pieces of her favorite blanket that she would take with her to school for comfort. My husband went from being a butt man to watching my ass contract and expand so much over the years and my boobs grow into enormous proportions that he frequently asks if he can have his milkies too. It's a joke but my boobs are fantastic. My three year old tries to nurse from time to time after watching his little sister spend countless hours attached to my udders.

As a stay at home mom I never saw the need except to curb the crying at the doctors office during those early visits. Always good to have around but I didn't use them. There are those moments where you have to work and transport and get ready and you don't have time to sit and feed and rock the baby so the pacifier is the next best thing. A piece of plastic that buys you time. If you are lucky buys you a nap too. With some distance from pacifiers I can tell you this, my kids both went through pretty big oral fixations. My son at 4 still bites and chews everything. I mean everything. Every toy, shirt, cup, towel, chair, you name it it's worse than having a puppy. Is it because I didn't use a pacifier? I don't know. Is it because I weaned him earlier than I should have? Who knows. If your baby cries a lot try swaddling and pacifiers. I used boobs and cuddling and walking around. I pack my kids up and try to take them for walks everyday. Anytime you can couple some exercise with sunshine and an activity that benefits and helps your children, it's all good in the hood.

28. Sex and the Scene of the Crime.

It would be much simpler and to the point to make a list of the things that don't go wonky with your girl parts during and after pregnancy. From a pleasure dome so enticing to your husband that he had to plant his seed into it to the Sarlacc in the Great Pit of Carkoon from Star Wars.

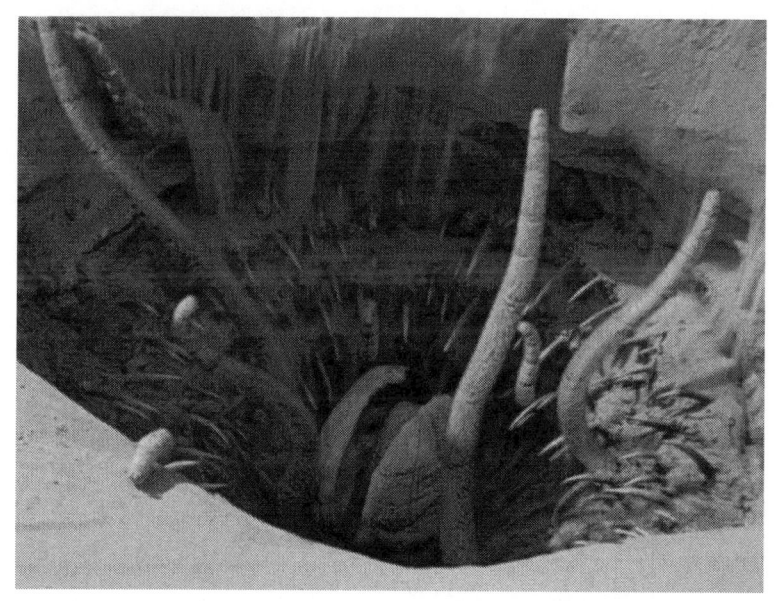

Movie "Star Wars VI: Return of the Jedi" Lucas Film 1983

Yeah that about sums it up. Do yourself a favor. There are dozens of lists of things you can and can't eat while pregnant, so read the short list of sex acts you shouldn't perform while pregnant and have your husband read it too to eliminate any heat of the moment accidents and so he CLEARLY understands what practices are off limits. Husbands tend to go in one of two directions. You are glass, they are afraid of you, they don't want anything to do with you. They are scared to hurt you, hurt the baby, that you are going to break, that their dicks are going to hit the baby in the head, please Tommy Lee I don't think so. OR they are so horned dogged out by having something strange that they are all over you. A good friend of mine who is very candid about sex and bragged how she couldn't keep her husband off of her. Her husband was on her all of the time while she was pregnant. A very petite girl who had always watched her figure and kept in impeccable shape gained 70 pounds. Her looks oriented husband couldn't keep his hands off her. Go figure. She went from dressing like Carrie in Sex in the City to a vagrant in her husbands old t-shirts and sweats. She also talked to me about the ups and downs of her sex drive before during and after pregnancy. Everyone is different. Most women feel like hot garbage. They stink. They itch. They ooze. Nothing they want to share with anyone. Some guys get very turned on by this. It's kind of like sticking it to a whale in my book. Now I always had the hots for my husband. I didn't worry really about hurting the baby while having sex during pregnancy. My husband kind of never broke routine and to this day it's always been the same. He does like me a little plumper from time to time so the weight gain doesn't effect our sex life, and when I'm in shape he's also DTF all of the time so I'm set. However sometimes an orgasm can trigger Braxton hicks contractions. That can be scary, uncomfortable and a little painful. I had a few painful encounters while pregnant. Mostly I just felt too big and quickly became out of breath. The best position by far for me while pregnant was doggy style. I'm sure your side could work too. I didn't want my husband on top of me but not nearly as much as he didn't want to take any chances with my belly or the baby. I have to say it was very business as usual except I felt big. Very much more of the same except that I was always a bit gassy.

There are some no no's during pregnancy and I'll go over them but if you can't stay away from these practices while pregnant really there is something wrong with you. Seriously. One is your partner, man or woman whatever you prefer, should not BLOW into your vagina while you are pregnant. Big no no. Don't do it. If it's part of your regular sex play then ooops you have to cool it for a while. Wasn't part of mine so moving on. Obviously find a position that doesn't crush the baby. No butt to vagina sex for bacterial and general health and safety reasons. I know there are a good number of you out there that like things very spicy and kinky. Now is just not the time. One you have a living human being inside of you and two you are going to be a parent. Maybe practicing some self restraint isn't a bad thing. Regular sex can be so much fun. Give it a try. Leave the latex mask and the 2 foot dongs in the bedside drawers for a while, and then make sure you child proof the hell out of that collection, or hide it where your little ones can't get to it.

Sex during pregnancy is like your eating. Sometimes you have crazy out of control cravings. You need it and you need it now. I felt that way during my last month of my first pregnancy. I was always fired up. My tastes have always been conservative so just regular sex please. But always. Everyday. All of the time. I will say it over and over again, being pregnant is kind of like being stoned all of the time. You are tired, you are hungry, you want like a burger, sex and a nap all at the same time. Maybe a milkshake too. Being big is not a deterrent to sex, there are ways around any issue.

I remember before marriage spending a lot of time grooming if I thought I was going to get lucky on a date or date night with a boyfriend. I would shower, very carefully wash up my lady parts, shave and then shave again, brush, floss, blow dry my hair, and do my make up to the best of my ability, sometimes starting over. I would spend time, a lot of time, picking out matching underwear sets, making sure the bra and panty went together if it wasn't a purchased set or even taking the tags off of something I had picked up at the local Frederick's of Hollywood outlet or bought on line. Then I'd pick out my actual clothes. How will these pants look with my bra when my shirt comes off. I would put on perfume, double check my breath, sometimes even double check my shave job in the mirror before I got dressed. Yeah, my husband stopped getting that a fancy presentation a long time ago and my doctor gets me gassy, with smelly lady parts, no shaving, swollen, and all kinds of nasty. Did I mention you lady parts will smell while you are pregnant? As do you feet, breath, you are all kinds of nasty funky stink and products you might ordinarily use to masks those unpleasant odors either make you sick or give you a headache and your nose is in super McGruff crime dog mode. The last thing you want while pregnant is a headache, especially with no real easy means of fixing it. coffee, umm no. aspirins? Ehhh yes but I didn't feel good about taking them unless I was really hurting for a long time. Cold soda, yes but in moderation.

Like it or not you husband gets a ton of unwanted exposure to some not so fun aspects of your poonanny. It's super exciting especially when you stink, are unshaved, and wearing some cotton granny panties that may or may not be stained and smell like pee. Lets not forget after your routine doctor appointments when you put those panties back on after having your doctors hands inside of you covered in KY, bring some baby wipes actually to wipe down before you get dressed again or you'll be goopy. I used the paper sheet they put on the exam table more than once to clean up with. It's not soft or kind to your parts, it has a wax coating so it doesn't do such a good job of getting lubricant off and if get stuck in your lady hair forget it. The paper also used to stick on my ass which would be not only sweaty but also have some lube and maybe some pee on it. note for anyone who's husband might still have some mysterious illusions about you, you might not want to have him see you picking pieces of waxed paper off your butt as you pull on those granny panties wiping down your cooch with a paper towel.

After 4 years of pregnancy with 3 deliveries and 2 babies my private parts are destroyed. They've had more damage than your body after a car accident and seen more trauma than your local ER. I've had dozens of stitches and I'm bruised, battered and scarred with nerve damage across the playing field. The birth of my son resulted in a handful of very carefully done stitches. I wasn't offered an episiotomy and told that they really don't do them anymore. I ripped superficially along the left side of my lady parts, from back to front. During the next delivery with my daughter the tearing of my lady parts went the opposite direction from front to back and I had a very sore butt. To this day I get phantom pains, I'll have an ache or even a stabbing feeling on the left part of my lady lips, its actually quite painful. I also have a chronic reminder of all of my butt stitches just in that the topography feels different back there and lets not forget the residual hemorrhoids that pop out from time to time.

Let's not forget while your lady parts are taking a beating, pummeling, a Rhonda Rousey level Mortal Kombat decimation, what is going on in the rear is just as traumatic. You butt takes serious damage. Hemorrhoids are just the start.   In the ultimate irony your body tests drive your skins elasticity and stretching ability by backing your colon up to maximum capacity then unleashing.   I found myself having to take a plunger into the bathroom with me most occasions, even when employing the drop and flush technique.   A sneak preview of just how something very large can be expelled from what seem to be very small orifices on your body.   I took a poop one night that was so painful and dramatic I almost called 911.   I was tired and flashing back to episodes of that show where they don't know they are pregnant so they think they have to poop and they actually give birth. After almost an hour of struggling I pooped out like a honeydew melon sized creation.   It was insane and again scary.

Your butt becomes like raw hamburger. The more you strain the worse the hemorrhoids get. The more you go and wipe the rawer your behind skin becomes. So in addition to all of the other irritants now your butt is on fire for 7 months. Enjoy. This is a great time to start using baby wipes if you didn't think of it.   After baby life is easier with baby wipes in all of your bathrooms and most of your other rooms too, but especially the kitchen and bedroom.   Your butt is going to undergo a transformation.   Not only will you probably tear, and probably tear in that direction so you are going to have stitches from your vagina to you butt, it just doesn't recover the way everything else does. Can I tell you I get phantom pain back there? Don't be embarrassed after baby to sit on ice packs and to have someone get your hemorrhoid pillow down at the drug store or better yet buy one before hand. Your butt takes a bigger hit than anyone will ever tell you and it's an injury that takes a while to heal and even then I still have loads of aches and pains associated with it due to I'm sure nerve damage and residual hemorrhoids and constipation issues. Buy yourself some Colace too.   It's over the counter but it is also what they give you in the hospital. You take it afterwards and talk to your doctor about what to take while you are pregnant.   You are going to feel geriatric. Incapacitated. If there is something available to help you then you might as well not suffer needlessly, there will be plenty of time to suffer later. Make yourself as happy and as comfortable as possible while you are pregnant. Be good to yourself, your body and your butt. The cherry on top of the sundae is that all of the crazy food you are craving is also going to get all Old Faithful on you and either explode out later or get backed up and store inside until you have a poop the size of a Fiat.

29. Stretch Marks, Leaky Bladders And Gas, Oh My!

You are dreaming if you think the usual suspects are the only physical symptoms you may experience. Morning sickness, nah, and actually I was expecting quite a few ill effects including back aches and gas. I got a few that I didn't even know were possible and you probably won't know unless you get them.

Just a sampling of some of your pregnancy and post baby body issues:

1) Leaks I smell like pee pees. Ooops. What? After the birth of my son I had a total loss of bladder control for 3 weeks. I called my doctor the week afterwards to say that I was peeing all over myself, all of the time. An after effect of giving birth and of the epidural. Drag. He said if it didn't get better in a few weeks we may have to talk about surgery. I did hundreds of Kegels everyday. Between nursing and doing Kegels my weight loss and exercise plan were complete. During my last pregnancy I had to wear panty liners from months 3 through 9 due to all of my daily leaks. I prefer Kotex panty liners, the thicker ones, or even Poise. They seem to stay put and absorb a lot without feeling too clunky.

The leaky bladder issues that had plagued me during the vast majority of my pregnancy were almost eliminated after delivery but alas in a reduce manner have settled in as a permanent part of my new body after babies. This is one of a few things that is starting to go a little haywire for her that my bladder even though I'm very healthy and in pretty good shape is really irrevocably altered. As much as I try to manage my pee pees, I often have leaks. I go before I leave the house, sometimes even twice before I go walk or workout. I go before I get in the car to go home if I stop off at my parents house or work. But the damage has been done. I find myself from time to time at the park with the kids after a long hike and I have a noticeable wet spot in my pants. I guess it just comes with the territory. I have a friend who always wants me to work out with her. She is a beast. Always going the latest and most challenging workout exercises. burpees, all that fun jumping stuff is off the docket for me. As soon as I try to jump or run for that matter my bladder releases. The Kegels don't help with that. It's just the way it is now. The new normal. I wear a poise pad now to play sports. I hide it by wearing multiple undergarments just to keep everything in place. While playing softball I wear a pair of running tights and a pair of compression capris over them. Then my cotton extra large panties and a poise pad. I tried just using an absorbent panty liner but I found that after running the bases I filled it up and it turned into a wet soggy almost like a water logged hot dog bun sitting in my underwear. Not a good look and not comfortable. I've had to accept the fact that I stink. I smell like pee. My house smells like pee. 3 dogs, 3 kids and a husband and no matter how much I scrub the floors and the toilets the house smells like pee. I smell right now. I just got back from a walk with my kids. Getting some exercise. I went to the bathroom twice before we left but the motion of walking up and down hills and jogging a bit to keep up with my 3 year old just jostled that urine right out of me.

2) Blockades On the opposite end of the spectrum is the fact that your colon is going to seize up. I woke up one morning 7 months pregnant at 2am. I felt compelled to poop. During my pregnancies I went from a once a day first thing in the morning person to a once or twice a week 'nuclear meltdown bring a plunger into the bathroom' gal. This particular early morning visit to the commode was scary and painful. I had to go. As I was on the potty my son woke up and tried to come in. I was crying. I was sweating. I was bracing myself up against the walls of the water closet. I tried to get him to go get his dad who was sleeping downstairs due to my extreme snoring. He was too young to understand. I labored in the bathroom for over an hour before something the size of a small baby came out of me. The whole time all I could imagine was those episodes of "I Didn't Know I Was Pregnant" where the girls give birth in a toilet. I didn't want my baby in the toilet. I almost tried to scrub it out with a toilet brush and sterilize the commode during one of my on and off times on the seat. I would crawl off the seat to writhe on the floor then back on. I tried walking around to loosen things up but ended up crawling. I was petrified. I couldn't make it far enough out of the bathroom to call for my husband or to get a phone. I almost reached in to relieve the plug manually. Almost. Bobby and Whitney time. I pushed so hard I thought I popped blood vessels in my eyeballs. I ended up delivering a 1-2 lb. poopie present. Yuck.

It's hard when your pregnant to eat the right things. If you follow strict dietary restrictions and ate properly you can greatly eliminate the blockage issues. However that is absolutely no fun and if you can't let go and eat what you want while you are pregnant when your cravings are out of this world and your enjoyment of food is at a super bong stoned level. You are given Colace in the hospital after you deliver to assist with your first poop. The fear that is put in you about how painful that will be is kind of bogus. I pooped the day after I got home from the hospital, so 3 days post delivery, and while it was a little uncomfortable mostly from the swelling around the stitches, it was fine. I bought Colace to have it home for the next delivery. Didn't need it. Went the day I got home, less than 2 days after delivery and even with a butt full of stitches it was no problem.

I have hemorrhoids that come and go. Stress, spicy foods, the moon cycle will bring about a flare. It gets worse when I exercise but can't get into the shower quick enough after. If I'm interrupted while pooping, yes it happens moms, little hands come under the door. Not matter how you try to mitigate the situation the kids know when you are pooping and try to light the house on fire. There will be times where you are going to the bathroom, and you think you have your kids secure and BOOM something goes awry and screams and all of that. In my case screams, dogs barking, crashes, nightmare. You don't get to wipe properly. You forget to come back and clean up or don't get a chance to for a while. That is the worst. That will make dormant hemorrhoids flare up like fireworks on the 4th of July.

3) Skin

You can use a case of bio oil. It's a crap shoot. Part genetics, part luck of the draw. You can't go wrong taking care of your skin and slathering on lotion but if it's your destiny then you are screwed. I gained a boat of weight. Lost it. Gained it. Lost it. A few marks but nothing major and I think they were from before I got pregnant.

If you do end up scared there are a few tricks. Try using some self tanner on the areas. It should make them more camouflaged. I'm sure a plastic surgeon somewhere has come up with a viable laser solution to diminish them that really works. Until then these are your battle scars. My mom likes to let me know at every possible point that I ruined her body and she could never wear a bikini after she was pregnant with me. If you do get crazy nasty stretch marks don't blame you kid. Your baby your choice your body. If your child isn't enough of a blessing to you then maybe being a parent isn't something that you wanted to do in the first place. One of the righteous joys of being an older parent is these kids are so wanted and so welcome and so loved. With out doubt without question. Many women now a days plan for a mommy lift to fix their belly and boobs. Set aside some dough to deal with your stretch marks too then if that's your gig.

Your skin does change. Mine is much itchier and drier than it ever was. Sometimes I think it's from the bio-oil, like lip balm which seems to have an overall negative drying effect. In the winter my skins dries out quicker and is prone to crack especially my knuckles, but that is from washing my hands a million times a day. Find a lotion you can live with, heck even steal from your kids stash.

4) Boobs

Again screwed. I'm finishing up nursing my 2nd baby in 3 years. I expect my DD's to shrink to a decent C and look like sand in socks in a few short weeks. Push up bra seems to be the best answer for those not into surgery. I was blessed to have smaller sized nipples. My boobs at 47 and nursing 2 babies over the last few years are decent. I might even take a picture. I would even dare say they are fabulous actually. Right now still nursing and slowly getting back into shape I love them. Another plus of being older is you stop giving a hoot about what other people think. I care about my own self worth, that my kids see me as a strong role model for self esteem and fitness and that my husband is satisfied. No one else exists in that equation. My boobs rock right now. They are big and juicy and functional and in a push up bra downright deadly. Shazam. They also itch. Right after I nurse I have a wet spot on my shirt and itchy boobs.

5) Frankenpussy

My husband says it's the same. I feel a few differences that could be babies, could be age, could be the massive amount of trauma over the last few years. Could also be the fact that with 2 kids your window to have sex is strange and odd and you have to be ready on the spot. I used to be almost always ready and I could get wet in an instant. Now not so much. It takes a bit for me to feel hosed down but then when I do it's major and almost too much. From Sahara to rain forest in a few minutes. Every once in a while I have phantom pains from I guess birth trauma and stitches. I find that all together sex is painful every once in a while, and it takes longer to get started, which sucks because we usually don't have a lot of time. You will feel me that first time you have snuck away to have sex and there are kids banging on the door or little hands and feet poking underneath the door and they are shouting and screaming for you. Nothing makes you want things to be over quicker than interference from your little ones, again ironic since that will make you tense up and make it harder to finish. Bugger.

6) Fart City

It's wrong. I'm sure you've been completely grossed out by a fart or gas cloud that your partner has laid down at some point. That does not compare to the unearthly toxic waste that your ass will release into the atmosphere.

7) Body by Pillsbury

Remember when looking at social media or postings of celebrities and princesses walking out of the hospital looking lean and fabulous that they have trainers, hair and make up and their livelihood depends on their looks so they work hard very hard harder than you will ever work to keep their bodies in shape. It's ok that you have a pouch and gained some weight and ate some donuts. It won't kill you. My take is that as long as your husband still wants to bang you it's all good. And if your husband loves

you it won't be an issue. I do look down with a bit of judgment on those who monitor their diets so stringently both during and after their pregnancy. Live a little. Enjoy those foods that taste so damn good while you are pregnant and fulfill a need. You have to give up every other vice you have so indulge just a wee bit. Men are not that complicated. If you married a man who has no problem commenting on your weight or says things to you like he's less attracted to you when you gain a few pounds then you might have some issues. If you married a cheater, good luck. Most of us are blessed enough to have married someone who loves us unconditionally and moving from being a girlfriend to a wife to the mother of his child only enhances his feelings for us.
Having said that however my body is wrecked. I work out hard. Harder than I ever have in my life and I'm vexed to get that scale to move and to get my body to firm up. I do want to get back into my pre-pregnancy clothes that are sitting in the back of my closet in space bags, sealed like a time capsule. I also can see how amazing my newer bigger hips and crazy big boobs are and I actually appreciate the juggernaut Kardashian social media phenomenon for helping reshape the concept of the perfect body. I know JLO really got the ball rolling but seriously to see Kim pregnant and rolly poly big I feel like yes this is what real women look like pregnant. When I see the other girls with big butts and boobs I think yup that is more realistic. Even though it's cartoonish it opens the door for a more grounded version of the female form.

8) Just let me whine for a minute

I have screwed up sinuses. A picture of health before all of my pregnancies now I have sinus issues. I get a raging headache right before it's going to rain. I have strange cravings still. Weird food combos enrapture me to this day. I have a messed up libido. I've got a perfect storm going on with that. I am getting older and technically pre-menopausal. I'm still nursing so I have those hormones. I have 2 kids rolling around. I have body issues.
My body creeks. Oh my joints ache. Like my sinuses right before it's going to rain my feet, ankles, knees, hips, lower back, shoulders, neck, elbows and wrists HURT. Ache. Make noise when I go up the stairs. My dentist who's known me for years

says pregnancy is like a disease that destroys your body. I felt ok and mostly really great during but some days now are absolutely brutal. Which makes me so crabby that the slightest situation that goes sideways or gives me stress can cause me to explode.

30. Good Luck with that Baby Weight, Bitch.

My hips are not going back to their former positions. This I've determined after trying for a year. Three pregnancies later they are stuck in an opened birthing canal position. I have a pair of juniors size 9 ripped very cool jeans in that bag as well as a boat load of sexy lingerie. Time to give it up. I'm lucky to be one of those women, well luck has nothing to do with it, I'm SMART enough to be one of those women who married a man who does like the way I look but loves me so deeply and respects me so intensely that my size at the moment isn't a concern, that little pouch of belly skin that might not ever go back right isn't on his radar, and the widening of my ass and hips just mean a bigger grip when he's hitting it from the back. I try to talk to him about my weight and he's bored, frustrated, even angry that I'm talking about it again and I need to get over it. Enough said. Thank you dearest husband. P.s. that's the way it's supposed to be ladies. If your husband has a problem with you 'getting fat' then start ticking off the days on your marriage.

My stomach is a mess. The skin is saggy and yuck and looks like cottage cheese under a layer of wet fleece. I don't think or hope it will ever look normal again either. My workouts would put most to shame. Two kids in a double stroller (~110 lbs) up big hills in my neighborhood for 45 minutest to an hour every day. Plus yoga, weights and core training. I can see a glimmer of definition under the flab. I feel like a jerk anytime I try to explain to people that yes I'm fit and I work out all of the time but I have this layer of flab on top that camouflages my buffness. Before I take a shower and without my glasses on in a dark bathroom in the mirror I look quite fit and fierce. Seems even more honest than the Photoshop techniques they use in the magazines. Like Leonitis in 300 I see shadows and definition and the outline of a kicking hourglass shape. I have big boobs, a little waist, nice shoulders and decent hips. Again, in the dark, without my glasses, sometimes the mirror fogged up from the shower I am supermodel. You better WORK.

Here is the irony. Nails and hair. Fierce. Boobs. Beyond belief. Even I sit and stare at them. They are amazing. Instead of a belly cast I want to take a boob cast. Once I'm done breastfeeding I know I will be left with sand in socks and have to put my faith into some serious push up bras but for now my tits are titiliciously amazing!! As my weight fluctuates because weight loss and fitness are not straight paths and I'm filled with the ups and downs of a mostly frustrating and sometimes rewarding roller coaster ride, my boobs get bigger as I gain weight. It's awesome. I can definitely distract how heavy my thighs are by highlighting my best up front assets.

Tracking my weight loss is like looking at the path of a cracked out rodent. Up, down, and all over the place. After my first pregnancy which did not end well I had gained a total of about 20 pounds. I was in ridiculous sick shape when I started, going to the gym 6 days a week for an hour minimum. My routine consisted of what I called the 'thousand'. I would start off doing two machines – at one weight below my max. I did 4 sets of 25 or 2 sets of 35 and a set of 40 for 100 total. I did them fast but correctly. I would then do 5 minutes of cardio trying to hit at least 50 calories burned. Then another two machines, doing 100 reps each, etc. until I hit 1000 reps and/or cardio calories burned. I was one of the first people at the gym every Saturday and Sunday when they opened. I worked out right after work and even before going out on a Friday night. I was into it. I eliminated all diet soda and bullshit substitutes from my diet. Went to brown rice, wheat pasta, all of that. What really helped was my husband. He was also realigning his fitness, reading a ton about how to get in shape and make lifestyle changes. He went to the gym with me even if we didn't work out together. I did a blend of girly stuff and men exercises. I did quite a few nautilus machines, also the squat rack and I really did not like doing cardio. Just not my thing. I had started at over 200 lbs. I'm a large framed person and yes I was heavy not just big boned, but I got my act together and got back in shape. Over the course of a year I went from about 205 to 145 then settled back up at 170 as my ideal weight. I was toned, decently low body fat, size 6 jeans and medium tops. The real casualty was my chest. I went from a 38D to a 34B.

So pregnancy One I went up 20 pounds. Those 20 never really came off. When I got pregnant I started giving into some food cravings and feel obligated to change up my fitness routine. I was playing softball 2 nights a week. Quit the team. They were mad but I wasn't taking any chances. Was playing tennis once a week. Stopped that. Went into the gym and you know what an absolute pain in the ass it is to cancel your membership. Uggh the manager who I knew decently well tries to talk me into putting my membership on hold. That way I don't have to pay the big initiation fee again. The on hold is only $25 a month. My god what a scam. They guarantee you won't be there and I didn't pay any initiation fees to begin with and didn't pay any when I joined again a few years later so don't just put your membership on hold, ridiculous. 2 months after I submitted the paperwork to corporate I finally got my membership cancelled. At the time you had to go in and have someone print a custom form that you sent in. I learned my lesson the hard way and sent it certified after there was no record of receiving it the first time. After that first pregnancy ended early I was craving to workout again. I started going for very long hikes with my dogs and lifting 10 pound barbells in my living room. I was just starting to see the results of my hard work over the last few months which had included running on a free treadmill we had in the garage. Running is not my thing. I'm a bigger person, my knees and joints suffer from it and it's just not my thing though the benefits are undeniable. 5 pounds down and just when I was ready to join the gym again, got pregnant.

Onto pregnancy Two which starts less than 3 months after pregnancy One ends. This time I put myself on restricted activity long before the doctors did. I wasn't taking any chances so once I found out I was pregnant, everything stopped. This was then exacerbated by some bleeding, the source was a uterine tear that delayed a much needed amnio to rule out genetic defects in this pregnancy. Once in the clear, and despite all of the advice to do light weights and keep walking I restricted my activity to prenatal yoga, and of course eating and sleeping. Here comes the weight this time up 60+ pounds over my starting figure which was already up from my fittest point.

I recognize how Jabba The Hut I got during my second pregnancy and I immediately resolve to get into shape. For first few weeks after having him I ate ridiculously healthy. My first meal was a salad and fruit. I kept that up for a bit. I had my son on a Friday, released from the hospital on Sunday and I was walking for exercise by Wednesday. Back doing weights by Saturday and decided to join the cheaper, $10 a month, gym in my area. I went 3 days a week to either do pretty long cardio and short weight workouts or I tried my hand at some classes including Zumba, Jillian Michael's Body Shred and Butt and Thigh Boot Camp. Along with some other factors including nursing I was back in a pair of pre-baby jeans at the 6 month mark. Brilliant.

The 6 months took its toll on me. Some emotional and family crisis saw me put my personal fitness on the back burner. I walked everywhere with my son in a front carrier, especially at night when I walked the dogs, but didn't do much of anything else. I gained back about 15 pounds. At the end of the year I changed gyms and tried to get back into the 1000 action item routine I had before I had gotten pregnant the first time. I even enlisted a workout partner and while she ran for 30 minutes I alternated between jogging and walking on a steep incline. I lost 10 pounds in less than 2 months and was on my way back and then, pregnant again. Same story. I put myself on restriction as this was the most hard fought for pregnancy of all as I wasn't sure I could get pregnant anymore. As an older mom you realize the days are ticking by so fast and every day you aren't pregnant is another day closer to menopause and not being able to anymore. So I stopped exercising except for yoga, started my competitive eating training, and gained 70 pounds over the next 9 months.

So here we are today, where I've been up and down and up and down over the last 5 years. My body has officially said screw you. I can't move the number on the scale for the life of me. A good day in my fitness world is 60-90 minutes of exercise including cardio, weights and yoga. And eating under 1500 sometimes under 1200 calories. That's a good day. String a few of those together and I can actually get some results.

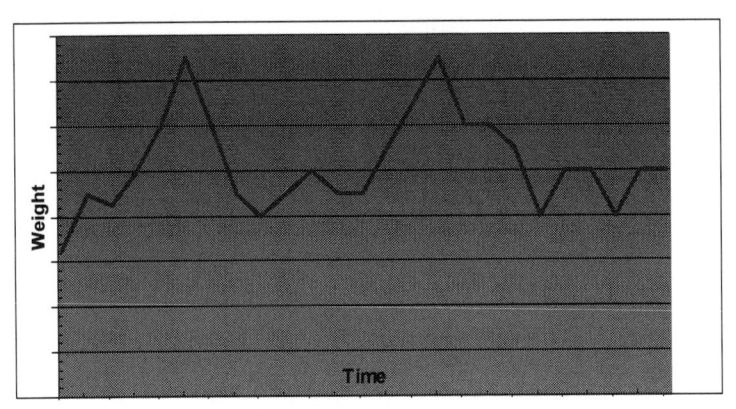

My weight gains and losses over last 5 years

The problem is the pendulum swings so wildly the other way. A bad day is eating 2000-3000 calories. Part of my nature is I'm always hungry. Always have been ever since I was a little kid. My mom used to take me to the buffet's at Marshall Fields (yes the department store) and I would eat SEVERAL servings of hand carved beef and mashed potatoes and ice cream. Never really met an all you can eat buffet I don't like. Vegas used to be my Mecca. Throw intense work outs and breastfeeding in and my normal unending hunger is a roaring raging entity unto it's self. Some days I can I can cap and I feel good and productive. But that one day I don't it undoes all of my work, weeks worth. The worst part of not being able to move the scale to be subject to these bouts, almost binges in the form of these very short lived fits where I can consume all of my food and calories that I wanted to eat for the entire day in a matter of minutes and that sets a bad example for my kids. So I'm not where I was before. I came about it honestly as they say. It's the lack of willpower that bothers me the most. For the past 5 years I've been pregnant or nursing or with a new baby and basically just tired with a house full of kids foods and snacks and being a stay at home mom I've learned to bake and cook so when I don't have something I want I make it. I've developed this gorging lifestyle to please myself at every turn with food since it was my only vice for the past few years. Is it me and my head? Is it my body protesting my choices over the last few years? I think it's a combination of both. My body is older and

I've put it through quite a bit the last few years. I didn't feel it then but I sure feel it now.

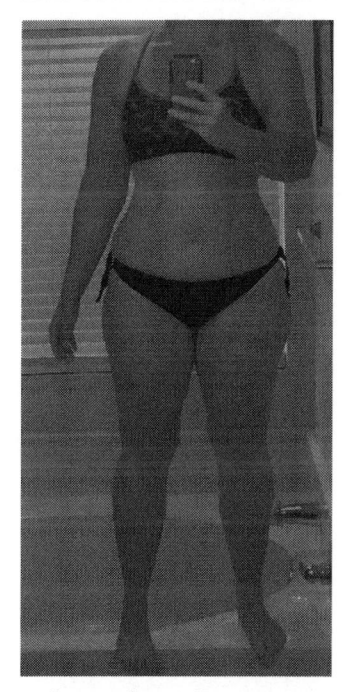

2 years after my last pregnancy

2 years now post my last baby and it's still a daily struggle. I mix up the routines, incorporate my kids, fight those no holds barred bad eating habits I laid in place during my pregnancies, do uphill 'death' marches with both kids in the stroller, lift weights on breaks and in the garage. As it would happen my hormones have also gone out of whack. Scourge of being older, I'm on the cusps of having the 'change' but still breastfeeding and not so far away from being pregnant for a few years straight so my body is a mess. But I'm fighting on. There is the cast offs to consider as well. The scraps your kids left and in my "clean plate club" mindset established by post great depressions grandparents I eat everything my kids try to waste and then some. Didn't finish that ice cream cone? No problem. Pizza? Sigh I guess I'll have to finish that too. The funny thing is I work out harder than I ever did. Except when I was an athlete in high school and running laps and doing sprints and drills didn't phase me, as an adult I know can put that memory

of childbirth as a carrot to dangle in front of me as I power through a workout and push my stroller filled with kids up a hard hill. If I did child birth and I didn't die and felt great afterwards I can do this I always say to myself. The knowledge that I want to be healthy for my kids and set the best example I can for them makes me push into workouts I would normally bypass for a snack break. Exhaustion makes you make bad food choices. It draws you towards sweets and junk food and away from things you need to prepare and are good for you. Who knows why. But it's true. It's all very Zen but for yourself and for your kids you need to learn how to master yourself and your mind. We study the philosophy of Bruce Lee in our house, along with the bible and the Phil Steele yearly guide to college football, and a few of the mantras Bruce is famous for are "be formless like water" "bend like a reed in the wind." It's just so hard to be mindful and stay on track on a daily basis. But I will continue to fight on.

31. Your Baby's New Home.

I love the Jewish tradition of not doing the nursery until the baby is born. Makes for a lot of work for someone, if you have a best friend or mother that will handle that you are in good shape. For the rest of us maybe that isn't practical. I like being prepared but in reality you aren't and will never be. Things will catch you off guard. I changed the configuration and layout of our nursery a dozen times after my son was born to try and make it more efficient.

You definitely want to designate an area before hand because you will start accumulating items. Boxes of diapers and general baby stuff takes up more room than you can imagine and you want to keep it semi organized and together. You will want to sort through everything you have to figure out what you might still need. Here is a hard piece of advice. Don't open everything. Don't wash everything. Don't take back your duplicates, yet. There is an overwhelming desire to have everything out, assembled, washed, hung up, and any doubles taken back to the store. Hold off for a few weeks. Target, Babies R Us, all of the stores that sell baby goods on a regular basis have very liberal return policies, even boxes of diapers that haven't been opened yet. You can take back almost anything months later without a receipt. If you can hold off and not open the presents under the Christmas tree until Christmas day your reward will be some savings that you can apply to diapers, wipes or clothes later. The clothes are the hardest part, you want to wash everything and hang it up so you can see it. You want to finish your nursery so it's all perfect. Do you best but if you can hold off and not take back that 3rd bottle of lotion you got at your shower, and not lay out 100 diapers into your diaper stacker, please do. You have no idea what your baby's true size is going to be yet and I felt very wasteful in having dozens of outfits that my kids never wore and ½ box of diapers they never used, and I did take back my duplicates for credit and it turned out a month later I needed that 2nd bottle of lotion and 3rd tube of nipple cream. You don't know exactly what you need until you are in a daily routine with your baby, and won't it be nice to have some nice a few weeks down the road to be able to take some items that you aren't using back for credit to get things you really want now that he or she is here.

A few ideas with notes on how to put together your baby area. Do keep in mind that in some cases, most cases, your spaces will all blur. My kids stayed with us in our room and in the kitchen / great room area. My son slept with me, my daughter in her bassinet then crib which was right next to my side of the bed. When the kids are little the placement is all about you. How do you function best. I've taken clothes and put them in and out of drawers and closets dozens upon dozens of time. Do you hang them up? Do you stack them in a drawer? I opted for a long time to keep a few outfits next to the diapers in the top drawer of the changing table and boy did I need them often. I still don't have it all where it works best for me. You want your key items as handy and convenient as possible. You need your diapers and wipes. We used a diaper genie for our first baby for pee pee diapers only. All poop went into a plastic grocery bag and straight into the garbage OUTSIDE. Don't leave poop in your house. Seriously. It will stink up the walls and carpets and you wont be able to get the smell out. For me I put diapers and wipes and bags in my top changing table drawer. Along with clothes, all of the clothes for the first month or so. And socks. There are days you will go through half a dozen outfits. You will be tired. You want everything handy. You want to spend time organizing. It sounds silly but spend a few minutes either each day or every other day restocking your diaper supply because you will desperately need wipes at some moment and you won't have any handy and the amount of damage you can do trying to grab wipes when your hands are poopie or the baby is poopie is astronomical.

I didn't do the big letters or anything fancy. I bought some white sheets for my son's old blue crib and a pink pad cover for our changing table. I didn't decorate at all actually. I admire the families that really put the effort into making their children's rooms perfect and decorated. Since I haven't done it in any other room in our home I guess it's just not my thing. Before my little ones I was over at the house of a friend of my husbands one afternoon. They had 2 kids with one on the way. Their rooms were perfect. Every detail and they were graduating their littlest who had just turned 2 out of the crib and into a toddler bed. They were going to need the crib for the next one. I happened to see the credit card receipt for this room transformation. It was over $2000 for just the bedding and décor. That didn't include the actual bed and mattress and furniture. I didn't spend that over the first year of my son's life including setting up the nursery and getting a stroller and diapers and car seats and all of that. Crazy. Sometimes I see the merit. As I'm currently finished with babies and my littlest is moving out of the baby stuff faster than I can stomach, I'm realizing even with my conservative stance I spent hundreds if not thousands of dollars on items that don't make it out alive or aren't any use to you after a certain very short period. I just put together a pack for a pregnant friend, actually a neighbor I've met once. In this pack is a breast pump, used only a few times, some clothes, a diaper bag and a monitor system. Retail about $500. I just want it to go to a good home. Between what you need to buy, what you want to buy, and holidays and parties and all of that it can get really pricey real fast. Does a one year old need a blow thousand dollar birthday party? My friend just had a carnival for her boys turning 4 and 5 which probably cost about $2000. Do you think the kids remember or it's the parents setting a memory and a milestone for themselves. There is always a reason to celebrate with kids and I'm perpetually on the fence about what is appropriate. I know I was raised to not celebrate enough, to not make enough of a fuss so if at 45 you want to throw your one and only baby the party of the century knock your self out! The results of some of us ladies having babies late in life is that they have a lot of resources to throw at it. The best of this and the best of that. In sharp contrast in some ways I feel blessed to be pretty broke and living in financial crisis mode for the last few years so I could stay at home. I live off my investments from years ago. I don't blow money. My kids don't have the best of everything, and as my son is 3 almost 4 we aren't lifelong Disney members and I've never taken them there. We don't have thousands of dollars worth of toys and clothes. But we have fun. We are cool. We love each other. I'm a home enjoying them and they are enjoying me every minute of every day. It's funny how many women are in my boat. Far more than I could have imagined. It's also funny how hard of a time I have trying to get new mommies together. You are on an island by yourself most days. Struggling to make your equation work. I never thought I'd be here. A full time housewife and mom. Are you kidding? Bitch I'm educated and an executive. Seriously. YES BTW. It's so awesome and if you can you should stay home at least for a while. It's a joy and a treat every single day. Today we did a bounce house, bubble dance party in the backyard. I bought a used bounce house, used my phone to play some mad fun tunes for the kids and a few dollars with of bubbles. Fun had by all and we often invite neighborhood kids over to play with us in the backyard. Beats the hell out of filling out TPS reports in triplicate.

32. Stay At Home Mom Guidelines.

I am currently a stay at home mom, which I never thought I would be. I thought before my son was born I'd be back to work in a week. I did work part time here and there. My husband was home and I'd work a few hours a week in the afternoons that first month or two. Then umm no. There is nothing more precious to me than being home with my kids. I love it. I'm constantly trying to convert other moms and dads over to the dark side with me. Sponge Bob is fun, better than watching the news. Hanging with the kids is a millions times better than going to work, and so what if you don't get a fancy vacation this year or tons of new clothes. Being with your child, and if you are super blessed children, everyday is a gift that should be cherished above all. It's exhausting, humiliating, wreaks havoc with your self esteem and sense of worth, is overwhelming but there is a laugh and a smile and a moment every single day that wipes that nastiness away and allows the sun to shine on your heart and soul. OMG barf, sappy but true.

Take a shower. Covered before but seriously, you will stink so take a shower everyday. It will make you feel and smell better. Also put on some moisturizer and a stitch of make up and maybe your hair in a chignon or a braid. You need to figure out how to follow this rule. Even if it means putting a screaming baby in a bassinet or crib for 10 minutes and going to the bathroom the farthest away so you can get a few minutes of peace. You need to shower. It helps you reset and clear your head from the clutter that the kids put in there. A baby crying and screaming does something to you as a person and as a mother. Its hard. It hurts. It fills your head and you can't think or clear it out until the screaming is resolved. What if it isn't. What if you have a fussy kid who always cries and screams. Its so hard to think. You are already muddy headed and this just makes you confused and quick to anger. The shower helps and it also lets you take a small break.

Get dressed. Try to put on an outfit that while comfortable and functional doesn't make you look like an extra from the wedding scene of Game of Thrones. Clean, decent fitting, which is hard to do those first few months. Nothing like a good pair of yoga pants, and I mean a decent pair, like go to Marshall's and buy a few pairs or better yet order some on line from Old Navy, their compression pants are awesome and can go a couple sizes up or down while holding their shape. Sounds very college but a zip hoodie is such a functional item. You need pockets. Your temperature will fluctuate especially if you are nursing. And a shirt that gives the baby easy access. I wear low cut tank tops. They are easy and functional and come in a ton of fun colors. Old Navy is your friend here, you can get your entire mom wardrobe during one of their spectacular ½ off seasonal sales.

I destroyed a dozen pairs of yoga pants in a few short years. I still have the pair I wore to the hospital last time which is a testament to their quality, construction and % of stretchy lycra. I had several pairs fail, one in yoga class ironically. I was about 7 months pregnant doing a pose and I looked down to find my pants had disintegrated at the upper right thigh seam. Barely holding together for a good 6 inches. That was the sad state of affairs with all of my yoga pants, which I threw away in groups after my last baby was born. They were stinky, stained, discolored and lacking inner thigh seam integrity. As a full time mom running around after 3 kids and 3 dogs I still am a yoga pants gal. I can however proudly say that I use them. I walk or workout everyday. I've watched enough episodes of What Not To Wear to hear Stacey London and Clinton Kelly in my had telling me what a cop out these outfits are. I've tried to make my gear look decent but at the end of the day it's a very unflattering mom uniform. There is a point where your parts and body doesn't go back and jeans aren't that hot of an option. They just don't feel good. The hips of them are too small and it's torture to get in them to then get a painful reminder of what once was. The back of your old jeans is too low and your butt crack peeks out. Your post pregnancy baby belly hangs out of the sides or over the buttons. The yoga pants provide good, flexible coverage and in their standard black color go with almost any top and provide a little camouflage. I recommend the high-waisted compression capri yoga pants from Old Navy. They are awesome. They stretch so you can wear them through a decent amount of weight fluctuation. They last through regular washing, without having to put them in the delicate wash or line dry them since you don't have the time or mental capacity to sort clothes anymore. They also give you some tummy flattening effects and hold everything in. Just buy new ones from time to time and make sure you don't have the see through version, yuck. You are also going to be insanely cold at some point during and after your pregnancy. You will want pockets for your phone and inevitably when you have little ones tissues and other necessities. Invest in a few pairs of pants and steal a big hoodie from your husband or partner while pregnant and do yourself a favor and get a figure flattering zip down the front and a little Michael Kors 'voodoo' hoodie with some color blocking and or shading that nips your waist and accentuates your goodies. It will make you feel better. Hard to go wrong with black on black. Looks sleek and appropriate on most occasions.

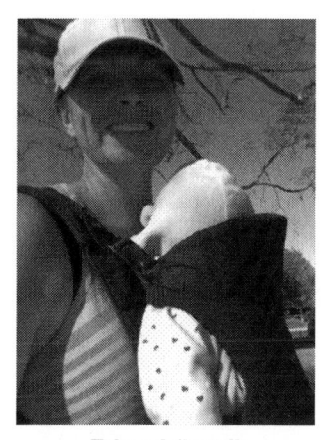

Take a daily walk

Stretch and do some exercises. You probably have yoga pants on already so do a little work. Walk up and down the stairs with the baby. Put the baby in a carrier and go for a walk. Stretch out your legs and back. There are tons of exercise options you can stream or record, and even if it's only 5 or 10 minutes, it will help both your mind and your body. Walking with a baby in a carrier is an insanely good exercise and a bonding experience all wrapped up into one. Get some fresh air and sunshine whenever you can. There is a reason people go crazy in climates where the sun doesn't come out much, you need it, it helps regulate your mood and for some women you might be home for a very long stretch for the first time in your life. You will see the dust on your baseboards and smell the odor coming out of your shower drains. Go for a walk to clear your head and get some sun.

Escape. Figure out what that is for you. My body temperature after babies is all screwed up. I'm always too hot or too cold and can't seem to be able to correct it quickly. I love going in my garage. Its always hot when I'm cold and cold when I'm hot. I'll stand in there for a few minutes pretending to find something. Getting my temperature straightened out helps me get my attitude smoothed over and helps me get a grip when things are going south. Some women like to lock themselves in the bathroom, I used to live down from a guy who hung out in his car for hours at a time listening to the radio. Find a place where the kids can't or won't follow for those times you need a minute or two.

There is no excuse for a dirty diaper. As a full time stay at home mom of 2 those diapers are changed on point. If I see a kid with a poop face we are going to get a diaper change. My children DO NOT sit around in nasty diapers. This is part of your job. I know you are tired. I know the last thing you want to do especially if you are sitting down for the first time in the day is to get up to change a diaper. Do it. it's not about you. For real. Wet is another topic. I do my best and change my kids as soon as I see a diaper dragging or they look full. No excuse for diaper rash as a stay at home mom. I try to change both whenever I can to just simplify my day so I'm not constantly changing diapers.

Make your own food. Buy the baby ninja and make food. Its so simple and worth it. They even have refillable squeeze bags you can buy. Make the food. Don't buy it. Make it. Why? Because you are someone's mom now. Make it with love. Make it so you know what's in it. It's not rocket science and no you don't need the baby food cookbooks. You use a knife. Peel a peach, pear, apple, cut up a banana, quick steam some zucchini or carrots. Put it in the blender with some liquid, formula or apple juice. Blend and feed. You will be deciding what these kids eat for the next decade, start figuring out what is best and what works and make it yourself. I cook every night. We can't afford to eat out but I also like to control what my family eats. Its so old fashioned and I'm not an old fashioned person but it's a priceless gift you give your family. With a 1 and 3 year old I just hit the point where we all can eat the same thing. It's awesome. Most baby food makers have these freezer storage trays like big ice cube trays really and you can make a weeks worth of food and store it then thaw it before you feed them. Think about the time it takes to go out and get food or buy food. You don't save anything. If you order dinner and you have to go pick it up, that is more time than I spend making a home made dinner for my family each night. Learn to make simple meals and your family will flourish. I'm not a gourmet by any stretch, but your kids only want simple offerings anyway. Grilled chicken, burgers, salads, rice, plain pasta. My kids get pancakes and fruit for breakfast. Takes about 5 minutes to make them a hot meal that they love.

Take care of the kids as best you can. Have them dressed and changed and fed. Play with them. Or throw toys at them while they are in their pack n play. If you husband or partner is like mine he doesn't care if I have the dishes done or his laundry done, my job is the kids. Period. If I get more than that done great. Kids, you, then everyone else. Good luck. It's tough. Everyday is a struggle to get it right. Some days are easier than others. Almost 4 years into being a full time mom and I feel amateur and stressed out most days. My good days are when my kids are happy and I have a good meal on the table, the house is clean and the laundry is done. My job before kids was never this demanding, difficult, impossible to master, full of variety, bringing new mental and physical challenges everyday. But my old boss never gave me that look and told me they loved me. Never cuddled with me on the sofa and asked 'mom are you happy?' to which I respond 'I'm always happy when I'm with you.' Kisses, hugs, falling asleep in my arms, soft warm skin and unconditional love. But it's still hard. Who am I to complain? Well I'm just your average mom with a lot of complaints about a lot of things and my day can go sideways in a millisecond. I love it. But it makes me so mad and angry and so frustrated I want to punch the wall. Mad that my kids don't comply, ha ha, and angry that I'm not always the mom and wife I want to be. It screws with your head man, the lack of sleep and the enormous serious responsibility of raising children. Do your best and tomorrow is a new day and a new opportunity to do it better.

Today we had a bubble party. For $12 I bought a big bottle of bubbles, bubble light sabers and a bubble camera. Every battery operated bubble maker we've ever bought has been a bust. Save your money. We had our neighbor over and had a bubble party in the backyard. We served some chips and Capn' Crunch in cups and had some Capri sun's to drink and blew bubbles and played music. Make a sanctuary for your kids. Make a couple actually. Places they can play and make a mess and you don't feel put out or obligated to clean it all of the time and they don't feel your stress for messing it up and being kids. That was a really hard one for me, how do I let them destroy things, and not lose my mind about it. I do my best to contain messes and have designated areas for it.

33. #TripleP-PukePoopPeeImmunity
Break Out Your HazMat Suit

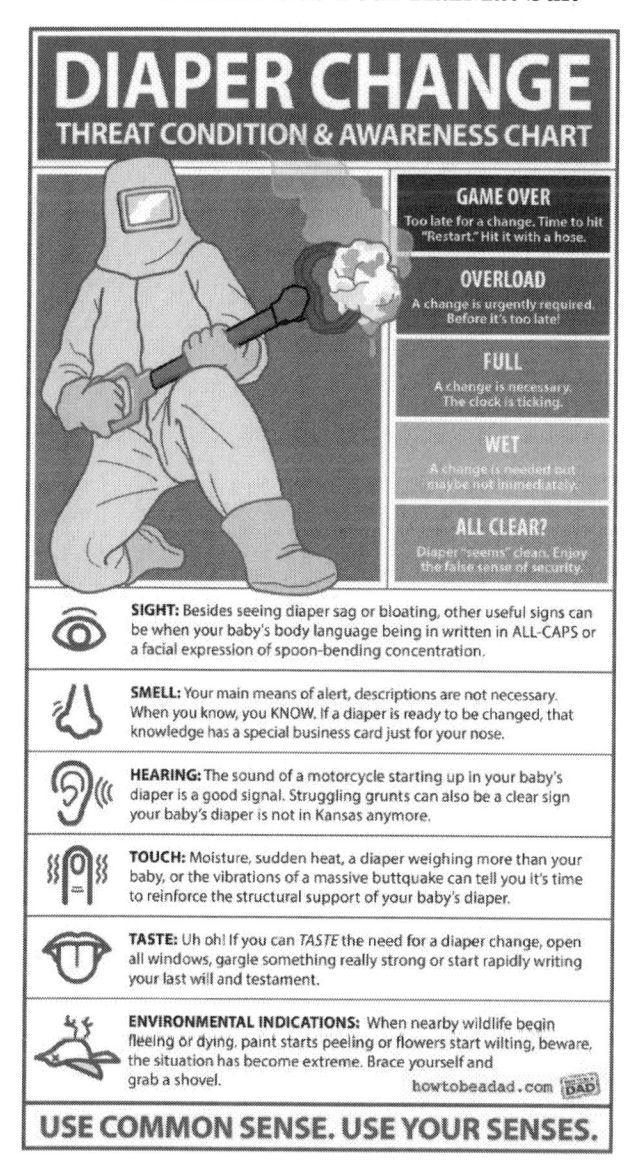

DIAPER CHANGE
THREAT CONDITION & AWARENESS CHART

GAME OVER
Too late for a change. Time to hit "Restart." Hit it with a hose.

OVERLOAD
A change is urgently required. Before it's too late!

FULL
A change is necessary. The clock is ticking.

WET
A change is needed but maybe not immediately.

ALL CLEAR?
Diaper "seems" clean. Enjoy the false sense of security.

SIGHT: Besides seeing diaper sag or bloating, other useful signs can be when your baby's body language being in written in ALL-CAPS or a facial expression of spoon-bending concentration.

SMELL: Your main means of alert, descriptions are not necessary. When you know, you KNOW. If a diaper is ready to be changed, that knowledge has a special business card just for your nose.

HEARING: The sound of a motorcycle starting up in your baby's diaper is a good signal. Struggling grunts can also be a clear sign your baby's diaper is not in Kansas anymore.

TOUCH: Moisture, sudden heat, a diaper weighing more than your baby, or the vibrations of a massive buttquake can tell you it's time to reinforce the structural support of your baby's diaper.

TASTE: Uh oh! If you can *TASTE* the need for a diaper change, open all windows, gargle something really strong or start rapidly writing your last will and testament.

ENVIRONMENTAL INDICATIONS: When nearby wildlife begin fleeing or dying, paint starts peeling or flowers start wilting, beware, the situation has become extreme. Brace yourself and grab a shovel.
howtobeadad.com

USE COMMON SENSE. USE YOUR SENSES.

Before babies my husband told me I would develop an immunity to all types of disgusting body fluids. I didn't believe him. Now with a baby, a toddler, a tween girl, a husband and 3 dogs my day is spent smelling, cleaning and identifying body fluids. My husband refers to me as the fart police as I frequently walk into a room and state "smells like farts." I've got a male Chihuahua who pees on EVERYTHING so I've got a superior scent detector and find myself picking up stuffed animals and smelling them for dog pee. I go through bedding doing the same thing looking for kid pee in the mornings, on the sheets and the pillows. This is your new life. It will revolve around peeing. A clock of pee, when they go, when you have to change a diaper, when the dogs go, when you go. Peeing all of the time. #PeePeeWorldDomination. While pregnant you have to pee, all of the time. It's like that time you were trying to get really fit so you drank a ton of water everyday and had to go the bathroom every hour or so. It's like that but so much more intense. It's preparation for what is to come.

A typical morning involves me changing two diapers, doing a sink of dishes, cleaning up any dog mess in the house, and throwing out the trash which usually has diapers and nasty used paper towels in it. This is followed by an array during the day of pee pee diapers and sometimes kid or dog pee pee on the floor and sofa. Cleaning the toilets out after my husband which is an industrial undertaking and I should hire a professional biohazard team. Picking up dog poop in the yard before the kids can run around and the whole thing usually starts all over again. While I'm changing the toddlers poo diaper the baby will puke and poo while in her walker getting the floor, her outfit, the walker, etc. While I'm changing the baby my toddler will help himself to something to eat and spill all over the floor. Milk and juice have a scary crazy spray btw, in need of Dr. Gil Grisom to identify the trajectory when dropped from a high chair or counter and can hit an entire 10x10 room including cabinets, chairs, baby furniture, anything in its path. I've found food and liquids on the dog's heads before. And you better get up every drop off of the floor and surrounding areas or it will get nasty sticky. While I'm cleaning the floor a dog will throw up or get scared by one of the kids chasing it and poop. After I get some sleep I'm going to start my own crime scene cleaning service. I've seen so much and smelled so much and had poop and puke all over me and all over my hands. The worst by far is explosive puke all down my shirt, all over the chair and the baby. The baby cleans up easy. It's the chair that takes a beating. That rotten milk smell never goes all the way away. Immediate hose down and scrubbing is required but the putrid smell will linger for months. Pouring vomited breast milk out of the cups of your bra isn't fun either.

I suggest the following; ***Alter your mindset about picking up spills and stains and cleaning up after accidents.*** It's a new part of your life you have to deal with so get used to it and try not to get mad or freak out. Your child WILL know when you have a new outfit on and will proceed to have explosive diarrhea all over you just to insure that you can never wear it again without some type of stain or smell to it. Your child WILL know when you have just washed the floors / scrubbed the floors / gotten on your hands and knees and done the corners and made the floors clean enough to eat off of. They will proceed to spill something of a foul smell or color in such a way that the CSI blood spatter pattern will encompass the entire area even under the refrigerator or stove. I had a kid once spill a bowl of oatmeal off of the highchair tray in such a manner than a few years later I'm still finding bits of it on everything from the wall behind the stove to the ceiling. It's like a slow motion summer blockbuster explosion and it's astronomical how many surfaces can be crushed and how much actual area can be effected. It's mind blowing that you can clean up after a five minute snack for an hour and still not be done. And while you are cleaning preparing for the other new norm which is they will get into even more trouble and make a bigger mess while you are trying to clean the first mess. It's reality. It's kids. It's maddening. It's frustrating. For a while it would make me so angry that every time I turned around or would spend a few minutes to even try to get ahead the kids would make me pay dearly.

Invest in the following:

> **A good stain removal survival kit**. This should consist of some type of spray or cleaning solution, cloths, and a spot-bot type handheld carpet / upholstery cleaner. You will use it all of the time. On chairs, rugs, mattresses, sofas, you name it your kids WILL poop, pee, throw up and get food on everything nice you own. Be prepared for doing some type of hardcore cleaning and

stain removal at least once a week. Sometimes sadly multiple times a day.

You might want to invest in a steam mop that converts to a handheld steaming device. It really makes everything feel very clean when you are able to steam it and then wipe it down.

> **Develop a stain removal routine**. You need to figure out a place to put your child that is out of your way while you are cleaning. In a pack n play or in their room but somewhere out of your way otherwise they will either make another worse mess or interfere with what you are trying to do or try to eat the cleaning solutions. I learned this lesson the hard way. All body fluid stains you want to deal with right away before the smell really sets in, so have a plan and learn how to act fast and not be too mad about it. I still get pissed off from time to time, as I'm trying to squirt out some Windex and the bottle is almost empty so it's making this pathetic noise and all that is coming out is a little white foam (sounds like my love life – haha) and I had just refilled it earlier in the week and you only have one pathetic little paper towel left on the roll because you've gone through them all in just a few days. A bad day will go through a roll of paper towels and other utility clean up towels and a few loads of laundry, breaking out the spot-bot, the mop and the vacuum maybe more than once all with a sink full of dirty pants or shirts. Don't forget to really disinfect or sterilize your sink after you wash something with poop out in it and PLEASE DO NOT wash poopie clothes in your main kitchen sink!! Especially over dishes. Like a fire drill or evacuation plan you need a poop drill so you can mobilize quickly and effectively when something happens and it always happens when you least expect it and you are ill prepared and exhausted so you can't think straight anyway. Do you want to get poop all over your house? Your door knobs, your sink, the floor, or yikes a rug. You will get it on yourself, it's inevitable. The more you can contain the situation, the better your plan the easier this nasty chronic chore will be dealt with. The closest bathroom sink is best and if you can transport in a plastic bag so it doesn't get everywhere.

> **Know what instrument is required for what spill**. A vacuum works best for food, cereal, anything dry and loose. Disposable paper towels for most body fluids and food, you don't want to transfer those things to your washing machine. Plastic toys can be washed in bulk in the dishwasher or sink with dish soap.

> **Alcohol**. Not necessarily on you and use extreme caution as some cleaning products will destroy certain surfaces but I alcohol almost everything now a days. I hate, loathe, detest, become absolutely sick and can't get the smell of bleach out of my nose for days so I don't use it. I use alcohol. It sterilizes, cleans and then evaporates.   To me it's the most friendly disinfectant and I utilize it to clean out the sink after I wash out poop clothes, I use it to clean up dog messes, and from time to time I use it to eradicate anything living on my counters. I hate the smell and thought of bleach so alcohol is my go to. Oh you thought I meant having a drink. I know those moms but a pretty strong aversion to alcohol in my early 30's, and trust me I drank enough for a lifetime, has left me on the outs with the cocktailing ladies. Coupled with pregnancies, trying to get pregnant, and breastfeeding having a drink hasn't been on my agenda for a very long time. But I say if your kids are safe have at it. One of the moms I know coaches her kids sports teams and regularly gets Costco sized bottles of booze as a thank you from the parents. Crazy.

There is such a biohazard feel about everything. A friend of mine described her disgust as a new parent feeling sweaty and stinky all of the time. Some of that is hormones, some is your body changing after baby and you do stink as your chemistry as been altered.   She completed the picture by telling me about having to scrub poop out from under her fingernails on a regular basis. I've tried dish gloves and disposable gloves but I don't like working in them at all as I lose the sensation of what I'm doing, I'd rather just scrub my hands down afterwards.

Notes on diapering. When your children are complacent and happy diapering is a breeze. Do it on the sofa, on the bed, my husband can change a diaper with the kid standing up on the counter.   So having your child pacified during diapering is like winning the lottery. You hope for it but it ain't happening. I have a changing table that is taller than normal because well I am tall and I want them at my level. I always, and I mean every frickin' time, do the exact same routine. When I don't things go haywire, and by that I mean diapers not on properly and either falling off, causing terrible chocolate leaks, or little red irritated rash points on the kids hips and legs.

First. Have your supplies ready BEFORE you start changing the diaper. I know you want to get it off and get the whole thing over with, but make sure you have your new diaper, wipes, a plastic bag for a poop diaper if necessary, a change of clothes and a towel or extra disposable changing pad all within reach. This is essential for poopie diapers, and especially when you are extremely fatigued. Spend a few minutes getting everything together before hand or it will go south on you quickly. I constantly stock and restock my supply areas during the week when I put clothes and toys away.

Second. Lay the child down on a surface that can be washed if necessary. Place the child in a manner that works best for you to work. I always have my kids with their head towards my left hand and their legs towards my right. Every single time. If I alter which way they are facing my brain to hand coordination gets screwed up and I start making mistakes.

Third. Slowly take the side adhesives off of the diaper, one at a time so you can evaluate the situation. If it's pee and you know its pee before hand you can be more cavalier, except with little boys who may have that cool breeze hit their boy parts and ignite their instinct to pee all over you and the changing area. In that case, keep them covered until you are ready with the new diaper. With pee, I keep the diaper underneath them, just in case they pee again or worse, start to poop, as I'm preparing the new diaper. I slide out the old one, and use my left hand pick them up by their ankles, hog tie style, and place the new one underneath. Tabs and elastic to the back and some idiot proof diapers actually say 'back' on them which is borderline handy, but tabs to the back is the best rule of thumb.

Third Step for Poop. Now when there is poop involved I make sure the wipes are open and within reach as well as a disposal bag that I hang on the corner of the top drawer of the changing table. I've got it down to 3 wipes. Maybe a few more if it's a total disaster and I almost never ruin the changing cover or get poop on my hands. Also assess the situation. Are the clothes effected? The pants are easy, you can check them as you take them off. Make sure the back of the shirt isn't soiled or that will get you and the changing pad. I always hold the feet steady and up by the ankles with my left hand. Some people like to wipe the bulk of the poop off with the inside front of the diaper as you slide it down. I always use a wipe to get the bulk of the matter and then deposit that wipe inside the diaper which is still underneath the baby. The 2nd wipe then does the outside area farthest away from me, then I fold it and do the outside closest to me. The third wipe does the final clean up and the butt. Make sure you search up their backside for poop. It can squish out of the back top of their diapers.

Boys vs. Girls. Boys sometimes get poop stuck in the little English muffin crevasses of their balls. Rub lightly until it's clean. Girls need a clean wipe straight down the middle, usually more than once. I do this the first time the wipe touches her skin so it isn't already soiled. Front to back with girls is the rule, and never ever back to front. You are asking for trouble with that. Take your time and get all of the poop. You know how you feel if you leave a little behind, it makes you itch and smell. Same for them, and add diaper rash on top of their problems. I make sure my kids are super clean and wiped down the best I possibly can before I put on a new diaper.

Fourth. With the new diaper underneath it's time to fasten and go. I use my right hand to do the tabs, first the farthest, so the baby's left side, then I take my time with the closest tab to make sure I have the fit correct. Diapers can get a little sideways, especially when your kids are wriggling and fighting with you. Depending on how I did I sometimes readjust the tab on the first side again.

There are different beliefs on where to put the diapers. A diaper with poop does not stay in our house. EVER. It immediately goes outside to the trash. End of sentence. The stink of having a kid in the house with a poopie diaper is enough, but leaving a poop diaper around will absolutely pollute any pleasant air in your home. It will become so foul you will throw up a little in your mouth. Pee diapers for us went in a diaper genie, then we gave up on that and the expensive replacement bags and just used a regular bathroom trash can lined with a plastic grocery bag that we take out every night.

Poop in General: Go until there is nothing on the wipes and their butt and all of the crevices are sparkling clean. You need to make sure every speck is off for a few reasons. One, if you leave but a trace it will smell and you will have to change and wipe them again to get that rancid awful smell away from you. Second, but a trace can lead to diaper rash, redness or itching and you want none of that for your precious baby. Also as tired as you are, exhausted, already in bed for some much deserved sleep or saddled up to a cup of coffee or plate of food in the kitchen for a much deserved break and snack, change that diaper as soon as you hear or smell it. Baby poop is a smell that can level cities and needs to be addressed immediately because an even worse smell is baby poop with air freshener on top of it, sitting like a sticky, sweet heavy cloud that fastens its self to the back of your throat and nose. Change dirty diapers immediately. It's not fun but it's your job so do it. At some point you will get poop everywhere. On the floor, the carpet, the sofa, etc. On you, and even one of my favorites in the TUB. A Caddyshack super special floater. Fun. The warm water can make them poop. If it's a turd consider yourself lucky. First take you kid out and immediately hose them off and rewash them in a different shower or bathtub. Set aside the towel you used to transport them in to be washed. Dress your child and put them somewhere so that you can work without them getting hurt and you being detracted for about 10 minutes. Now get a wipe in your hand and gloves if you want them and get that turd out and flush it down the toilet. Drain the tub. Fish out any toys. If you are inclined to save them put them in a sink and super clean sterilize them with hot water and rubbing alcohol. Some toys won't stand up to that level of cleaning, so be it and throw them away. Clean the tub, wipe it down with rubbing alcohol and make sure you cleaned the drain well. If it wasn't a solid poop, well just throw away everything that was in the tub or set yourself up for defcon 5 level sterilization, and again clean the tub. Use paper towels so you can throw them away. Not a fun job, one of the worst, but it needs to be done and be done immediately and you don't want any poop or bacteria lingering on anything your baby will touch, play with, or put in their mouths later.

The bottom line is that as a stay at home parent, or even a new parent in general, your sales goals are replaced by poop and pee. You will be willing and able to tell anyone and everyone, whether its appropriate or not, how many times a day your child has gone to the bathroom. I have had my sister shoot me a look over Thanksgiving family dinner to STFU when I start talking about my kids going poo or pee. She is so grossed out by it, I'm just a 'breeder' in her eyes. Haha. Forget about it when it's potty training time. Your focus is on their bathroom functions. Period. I want to tell everyone that my son's new technique for pooping, as he's figuring out when he needs to go and how to get it all out so he doesn't have to go again a few minutes later, is to climb on the bowl so his feet are on the seat and squat. That way he can kind of see what is coming out and that gives him some sense of accomplishment I guess. #PooPooGoals. This is after being fascinated for over a year with poop. He used to ask me to show him his poopie diaper and measure whether it was a 'good' poop or a 'bad' poop. All poops are good I'd tell him. His obsession then turned to the bathroom, the water closet as it were. He's tried going without putting the seat down, yuck BTW because he grabs the inside of the rim which after being in our home for 10 years is the one part of the toilet I can't get super clean. He also had a phase where he turned backwards so his feet faced the back wall, still grabbing the inside rim, no seat, cowgirl style.

When it comes to body fluids let's not leave boogers off of the list. Are you kidding. They see you coming when you want to help them get rid of them. As soon as they turn the developmental corner and they can get them themselves you are really in for it. Boogers everywhere. On clothes, in their hair, on the chair, on your hand. I have kids who are pretty darn healthy with the odd cold here and there and snot seems to be the wild card. What to do with it? I'm nursing and look down and my boob is covered with snot. I always ends up with a handful and never a wipe or tissue to put it in. With little ones who love to grab toilet paper like it's a ticket tape parade I find myself without any options for boogers outside of using my shirt. Yuck. You've also never experienced the juggernaut type strength children from 3 months to 3 years can exhibit when you want to relieve them of a mucus or booger problem. You feel like you are going to hurt them just trying to clear their noses.

So suit up, get your gear ready and seriously invest the time into figuring out routines that work best for you because you will be dealing with fluids and messes and disasters day in and day out and the more you can contain the crisis through preparation and preplanning the more sanity points you will retain at the end of the day.

34. The Stickiest Of the Icky. 2x The Kids = Clean Up x 100.

Before babies my house was ok. Now it's pretty f'ing clean. You can literally eat off of the floor. Even at that it will never be perfect. While nesting I found I had not only super smell but bionic vision and Donald Trump levels of disgust for all dirt and dust. You need to get all Frozen on it and 'Let it go.' Let go of your desire to be super clean. To not be sticky. Get really good at doing spot treatments and patient about having the clean the same spot on the floor over and over and over again. Its maddening but the reality is you are going to be in a non stop cyclone of dishes, laundry, floors, bathrooms, kids, etc. The amount of tasks you have as a stay at home mom on a daily basis is daunting, and makes you wish for the simpler days going into the office with a 5-10 item to do list. Hell I do that during the first 10 minutes I'm awake every morning. You hit the ground running. You have kids who immediately need to be changed, fed, cleaned, and will make a mess bigger than any mess you are trying to keep them away from while you are cleaning.

As a kid I used to watch the Love Boat every week and how glamorous did I think Julie McCoy was for being the Cruise Director on the Pacific Princess. That's what being a mom is like. You are the Cruise Director and it's an awful job. All everyone does is complain and every day starts a new that you have to fill with food and activities. What a drag. Seriously though that's what it's like and it does require some discipline and structure. I tried to free form things with one kid but once I had two little ones in the mix a routine becomes necessary or you'll never get out of the kitchen and off the changing table. The mess and chaos and the time spent dealing with that will far out weigh the time you put in trying to create order and a schedule. List of activities. Not shuffleboard but outside play time. Not a mixer but how about a play date and bonus at the park. We also need exercise and instruction. It's no joke, its hard work and every day brings a new set of challenges and as soon as you get traction with a routine it will change either because the kids are growing up or because your needs are changing.

Our current schedule is as follows and I know it will be different next month:

Wake up.

Start the coffee.

Feed the dogs. Have a sick dog so he needs a set of medicine.

Feed the hermit crabs the kids talked me into for their birthday this year. Make sure they are all still alive.

Make my husband's lunch.

Straighten up downstairs, pick up all dishes, trash, toys.

If baby is up, she gets breakfast number 1. Fruit and a drink. Start setting aside food for toddler breakfast.

While baby is in high chair try to put dishes away. If time permits fold laundry at counter. If chores are done stretch and do some wake up exercises.

After breakfast 1, baby gets diaper and clothes changed.

If then toddler is up turn on Disney TV for him, take him to the bathroom to go pee pee. He is toilet training so then put him in a training pant and change his clothes.

Set toddler breakfast up, baby gets breakfast #2.

Second round of kitchen cleaning. Counter and surfaces wiped down.

Address any laundry and dishes.

Add anything we need to our weekly grocery list. Plan dinner.

Get ready to go for a walk if weather permits. Get 2 drinks and some snacks. Clean off stroller if necessary.

Get dressed to go for walk. Everyone needs socks, shoes, and baby needs a jacket if it's chilly.

Go for a walk. Stop at a park to play.

Come home for lunch time. If baby is asleep bring her in and let her nap. If not set up lunch.

Assemble lunch. Turkey, cheese, apple and crackers. Juice in sippy cups.

Wipe down kitchen and kids.

Put dishes in the sink for later. Hope it isn't overflowing yet.

Shared bath time.

Try to keep the water in the tub, the chaos down to a minimum. It's very Noah's arc some days where I will end up with a full blown flood on the bathroom floor.

Get a few minutes of writing done. The big bathtub is in our master bedroom so I can see the kids from my computer desk. Pay bills, answer emails, while the kids play.

After baths get kids dressed again, put on show and jump in the shower myself real quick.

Quick shower and dressed.

Afternoon play time downstairs. Put on Nick Jr. Do some writing, drawing, building.

Clean up the dog poop outside.

Change a poopie diaper, help my son go poop in the potty.

Outside playtime if weather permits. Play dough is always a winner and running around in the backyard.

Workout if kids permit. Try to stretch and do some light weights while the kids are in the backyard.

Get house straightened up and things ready for daddy to come home.

Prepare and serve dinner.

Put away laundry.

Do dishes.

Clean kitchen.

Get the kids to sleep – yeah good luck with that.

Get ready to start over tomorrow!!

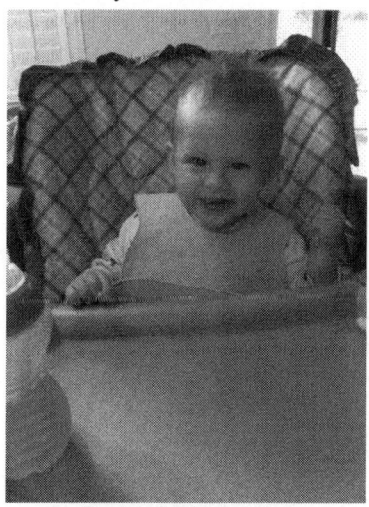

Jacob in his high chair

Call it the doldrums, call it monotonous. There is never enough time in the day to get done what you need to do. As much as you want to be organized and treat it as a business, boy that sure takes the fun out of it. My husband is an amazing father with the best point of view on all of it. He says let the kids be kids. When the news has to run reports on over scheduled children having anxiety and not sleeping well you know its pandemic. I have an agenda for the day or the week. Sometimes I hit it all, sometimes I don't. When I hit it all I make a new one. Schedules and to do items are like laundry and dishes and cleaning the bathrooms. You gotta do it but it never stops. Ever. And if you let it rule your life what fun is that for you or the kids. Being a stay at home mom is about cleaning and organizing but it also needs to be about being flexible and ready and not putting on so much pressure on everything that you miss out. What is the point of sacrificing to be at home if you don't enjoy it. If it's all arduous then you could have someone else do it easy enough.

35. But It's Supposed to be About ME!!!

Yeah. Kiss those days goodbye. In theory many women and couples try to create time for themselves and spa days and date nights. I respect and am jealous of all of that. I never understood spa days until I was 2 kids deep with post pregnancy issues and chasing toddlers around generating aches and pains that won't go away and a total lack of any decent sleep leaving my body crying for pampering while my mind is craving the silence and tranquility of having a child free afternoon. Date night, same thing, need time to get away. The reality is however you will NEVER stop thinking about your little ones and wanting to put them first. I have no problem putting myself on the back burner to do everything I can for my little ones. As I'm getting older I do realize I need like 10 minutes to shower properly but that usually involves having someone else in the bathroom or even in the shower stall with me, whether it's a kid or a dog, and I don't have any privacy. If I lock them out for a few minutes they beat on the door and holler and scream until I let them in, and little hands and feet make their way through the gap under the door.

I do try to look my best, especially if I'm leaving the house. When I know I'm going to be home with the kids all day I do a little make up, a little hair, decent clean functional outfit. Yoga pants baby and a tank for easy nursing. I gave up on nursing bra's a long time ago. Mostly because I accidentally either washed or dried them too many times and they were falling apart. Also my fluctuation cup sizes with dieting etc. and the kind of poor construction of most of the bra cups made them impractical. So I use a regular t-shirt bra and just pull the cup aside. The shirts however are the key. Need something lower cut with access that won't get disfigured by being pulled side over and over again. I don't like the whole pull the shirt up thing. Yuck. I have no desire to expose my belly like that. My boobs yes they are fabulous, belly no. Feels too uncomfortable. So yoga pants for speed and ease of movement, a regular t-shirt bra with formed cups and underwire for shape, a nice tank t-shirt or workout top and hair in a pony tail or bun. Trust me about your hair. You want it UP as much as possible. Those little ones will RIP IT OUT every chance they get. Same with jewelry, maybe a wedding ring but a necklace is a noose and earrings are just shiny things they want to grab and rip out. Nothing funner than getting punched in the eye, pooped and barfed on, nipples bit and hair ripped out all at once. Add dogs into the mix and having the occasional accident in the house and it's flipping PooPooPeePee-O-Geddon.

No it's not about you anymore. Not even close. Did you think it would be? I go out with my husband and I have triple the amount of stress and anxiety about how the kids are acting for their grandparents then I do when I'm home. I love my husband, I love my kids, my husband loves me, he loves our kids, we'd all just rather be at home with each other for now. Especially while they are little. Its easy and blissful. I'd rather watch my kids play for hours on end than do almost anything else on this planet. I don't see the rush or the need to go out and be alone. Does it make you better parents? I don't know. I feel that from time to time you do need a break so you don't hurt yourself or your kids when all of the stress piles up and things start going avalanche wrong in the course of your day, like the 5th clothing change, or slipping in dog pee or just now my daughter stepped on my foot which caused me to flinch back in my chair and my son had put a bunch of crap on the floor building a fort so the chair caught it and toppled backwards with me in it and I may have just hurt my back and pulled a muscle in my gut and I want to scream and yell and grab and I have to take a breath. Having a sanctuary inside the house would probably work better then forking up the hundreds of dollars it costs to hire babysitters and go out for a date night. Remember the old "Calgon take me away" commercials. You need a few of those moments everyday. Ones where you know the kids can't get hurt, and when you've gone beyond caring if they make a mess or destroy something you just need a break.

I wish I had more mystical sounding take but you decided to be a parent so for now, and who knows how many more years in the future, you are in charge of someone who cannot take care of themselves. So no, it's not about you or your husband it's about them because they are incapable of meeting their own basic needs.

36. Ever Changing Moods.

The sleep deprivation its self is a serious mind screw. So let's add frustration, exhaustion and self doubt on top of it.

Crabby beyond all recognition. Having a baby fixes nothing and just adds tremendously to your stress and problems. You think you are pissed at your husband for leaving his dirty clothes on the floor now? Wait until that baby comes and he doesn't even budge or offer to get up for night feedings and you haven't slept in days and the baby is fussy and won't stop crying and you trip over your husbands clothes or shoes that he's left in the hallway or on the floor. You will go nuclear. You will say things that are divorce oriented. After changing diapers and throw up and those days were the baby is just out of sorts and you are out of sorts, and you've been peed on and pooped on and thrown up on and then right after you clean up and change you are clumsy and spill coffee on yourself, cleaning up after your husbands "taco Tuesday with the boys" toilet explosions are going to warranty a call to lawyer or an order of protection for your husband by the local police. I want to yell from the rooftops, I want to smack my husband, I want to get all scientology on his ass and make him scrub the bathroom on his hands and knees with his own toothbrush. But I remember that this was my choice. I chose to have these kids and opt out of the rat race for a while and be a full time stay at home mom and wife.

Daily decision making more intense than your latte order at Starbucks. It's an odd role for a former executive. One I'm ok at, not great, not awful, just ok. I see loads of other Pinterest mammas who are so super organized. They always have snack bags for the park. The kids are always dressed right. They have activities and crafts and learning sessions planned all day everyday and their kids are clever and well behaved and the moms are always dressed nice and their hair is done. That isn't me. With all of my smarts and education that is not me at all. Everyday is a crisis, one I try to manage better and better but I'm struggling, hustling from one meal and one diaper to the next. I distinctly remember a day I forgot to feed my son lunch. No lunch. I was pregnant and just struggling to stay on my feet and awake and running after him and I didn't feed him lunch. Now you say didn't he pitch a fit, wasn't he crabby. No he is the kid that isn't that food oriented and I've been so loosy goosy with that we didn't really have a schedule or a lot of structure in our day and I would feed him all of the time, every free minute when I would think of it I would make him a snack or a meal and hoped he would be enticed to eat. I missed a whole meal one day. I've made that mistake once or twice since then, usually with dinner and usually though when he has taken a late nap and woken up in the evening or something to that effect. Diaper to diaper. Did I change her diaper? When? Should I again? What if she gets diaper rash? What if it leaks onto the sofa, floor, bed? Did she eat breakfast? Was it enough? Damn I went a whole day without getting her to eat greens. Did I brush her teeth? The complexity of child care while it seems simple is a day filled with tasks, chores and decisions. It's rough. Then if you want to be super mom on top of it all you need to do all of the planning to teach and have learning time and imagination time and play time and craft time. I'm not that mom who gets on the floor and plays. I'm not that mom who spoon feeds the kids. On top of all of that what about the super wife stuff. House clean, dinner made. More tasks. More decisions. Being a full time working executive is a walk in the park compared to this. As a long time single woman just taking care of myself was challenging enough. Let alone now a house full, with a husband, 3 kids and 3 dogs. Those poor dogs. Not only do I completely neglect these poor animals who haven't been walked in over a year, thank goodness for our nice yard and that they are small and old enough that they don't need to walk too much. I don't get much learning done. It's either ABC's or dishes. 123's or dinner. The popular phrase is Beyonce has 24 hours in a day just like you and look what she does. She does it with trainers and chefs and nanny's and assistants. I'm all alone here.

37. When I Get Some Sleep.

Having babies over 40 does have some serious drawbacks. My body hurts. My ankles and knees are destroyed. Those hormones that surge through your body to loosen your ligaments and allow the parting of the sea for the baby to move through your birth canal do a right smart job on any old sports injury. They settle into joints, wrists, knees, ankles, etc. My belly is not going back without surgical intervention. Everything hurts and this is magnified by the lack of sleep. I keep putting things off until I get some sleep. That may never come. Or at least not for quite a few years. I'm so tired all of the time and my body hurts. It's hard.

However then you factor in the advantages of having babies over 40's. There is a very small chance it's unplanned. I say to myself everyday how lucky and blessed I am to have two happy healthy children and how I have defied the odds and statistics. Even while pregnant and feeling miserable I did my best to suck it up. This is what I wanted. It's temporary. Being older allows you to take the Phil Jackson Zen approach to your daily stressers. This is what I wanted. I'm lucky to be in this position. It's all temporary and in the long term I'm manifested my dreams. I'll miss it when it's gone. Currently I'm nursing my 10 month old baby. She has four ginormous horse teeth that she loves using to bite me. I'm afraid she's going to bite my nipple off. My totally desensitized boobies are screaming in pain when she clamps down like a frickin' pit bull. I wince. I yell. I tell her to stop. I cover up. I tell myself this is it. Time for a bottle. Then I reconcile this is it. I will never have this again. It all moves so fast. For the years I felt I was sitting in idle not doing much of anything this time is screaming by and I can't get enough sleep to catch up and enjoy it.

Tired. So so tired. Sleeping and napping while pregnant is such a sweet blissful act. Your body is so preoccupied crating a new life that it gives you a free pass to sleep as often and as long as your schedule allows. It's an evil irony however making sleep so intoxicating and delicious while pregnant to violently rip it away from you after the baby arrives. Almost 4 years into having children and I have had maybe 10 solid nights sleep. You can't even savor it when you have one. You wake feeling disoriented from sleeping too long and actually dreaming and its gone in an instant. Feels like you just laid down. I don't have the answer. I don't know the secret. I have a one year old I'm still nursing and when she fusses at night I nurse her. I guess I'm supposed to let her fuss. That doesn't work for our dynamic.

Most days it's overstimulation city. I find myself having a short fuse and losing my patience to the most ridiculous reasons. The kids are all over me. Poking me. Touching me. Pinching me. The little one digs her fingernails into my boobs while I'm nursing. The older one used to pick or any beauty marks on my chest, until the bled, and screw around with my bra straps. I don't get a minute to have a proper meal, uninterrupted, sitting down, without a kid screaming or pushing on me. They know, yes they know, when you are on the phone or need a moment to yourself and that's when they go into overdrive. As I'm typing this book my little one like to ram her head under my right arm, and then with great effort get into my lap so she can hit all of the keys. It's maddening. I can't even move my fingers to type because she's squirming and screwing around. I tried to eat a bite of lunch today. Standing up. At the counter. Nope. She had other plans. She butted her head onto my legs with such force that it knocked her back into the kitchen cabinets and pushed me away from my plate to where I spilled my forkful.

Madness? THIS IS EVERYDAY PARENTING. You never get any sleep. You have to figure it out. How to turn off your overly sensitive sense of feel when they are crawling all over you and you just want a moment of peace. You have to turn off those overly sensitive ears when the screaming and the crying starts. How do you put a thought together or get something done when it just never stops.

38. Waylaid By Jackassary.

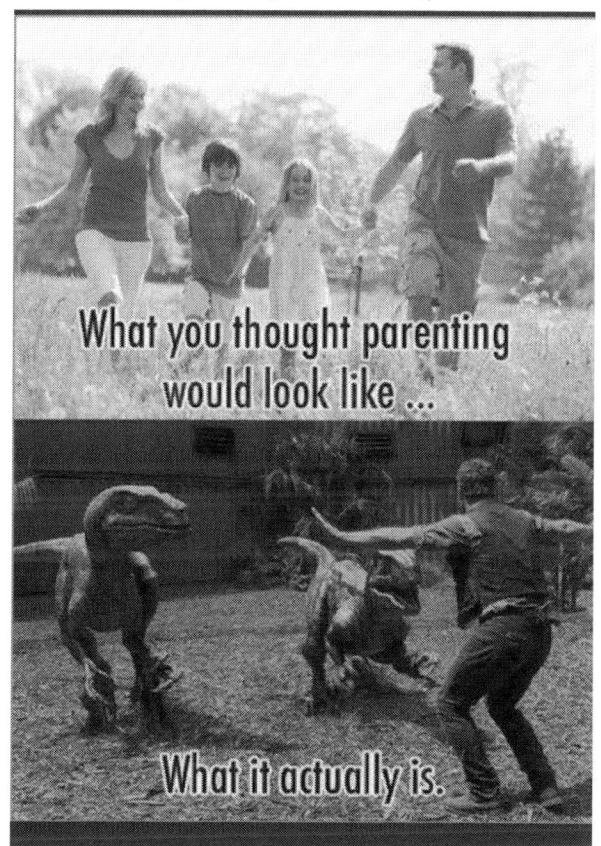

What you thought parenting would look like ...

What it actually is.

Movie "Jurrasic World" Universal Pictures 2018

Welcome to parenthood. It's all jackassary. Except its being performed by drunk little monkeys. I cannot tell you how infuriating it is to have a daily struggle with my children on the simplest of tasks. Changing a diaper and dressing them are Olympic trials. My littlest likes to flip while I'm changing a diaper or bang her fists like King Kong on her privates while I'm wiping up poop. I'm embarrassed to say that I found my older boy uttering a phrase around the age of 3 that made me absolutely mortified, he said more than once, "Get you fucking foot in there." Are you kidding? I had NO idea he was retaining that. When the fates have dealt you the non-cooperation card for the day it can be brutal. Before kids could you ever imagine losing your cool because a little baby flexes her foot when the pants are going on making pulling the pant leg on nearly impossible. Where was this information In Physics class? This seems stupid and trivial but one of the overriding issues you will deal with as a parent is trying to get a leg into pants, a foot into socks (oh that is the worst), arms into sleeves, and feet into shoes. They flex and contort to make the chore near impossible, sometimes to the point where you are forcing their limbs, others where you give up and have to start all over. The getting dressed struggle is real. They move and angle their hands and feet so you can't get their pant legs on, their toes grab and feet tense and halt the progress of the pant leg and you can't pull them up. Start over. You have to scrunch up and accordion the pant legs to get them on. Same with the sleeves. They hook their hands and thumbs on the inside of their shirt sleeves in such a way that you just have to start over 'cause it ain't going on. My favorite is when you are all sweaty and at the end of your rope from fighting with them for a few minutes to get a diaper, pants, shirt on them they start taking something off as you are putting another thing on. When they figure out how to unfasten diapers, good luck. You are wrestling with them to get a shirt on and they are bent over undoing their diapers.

Now diapers are no joke either. When they don't want to cooperate it's apocalyptic. On a bad day, with 8 diaper changes which involve pants coming off and on and usually a total clothing change or two, it can feel like all you are doing is struggling with your child. I find myself so angry and exasperated sometimes just trying to keep the little ones from putting their hands in their own poop while I'm trying to clean them up. Oh my God, they squirm and wiggle and sometimes it gets very WWE and I feel like I'm putting a choke hold on the little ones just to try and get a diaper on them. I do my best to keep our changing area, my child and myself poop free but it doesn't always work that way especially when they get it in them that they are leaving, moving, getting away. I feel terrible when I place a strong arm down across my little ones, while I have a grip on both ankles so I can clean the offending area, at the same time trying to keep their little wandering hands away. My girl is a born helper so she wants to help mommy wipe up her parts. My boy is a clown, it's clown school and once he gets a taste that his antics rile me up or get under my skin BAM he's amplified 100%. Nothing more exhausting than being tired from lack of sleep, having a non compliant child and doing everything in your power to bend like a reed in the wind to keep from getting poop on you. I've gotten to the stage where I don't do poop removal from clothing anymore unless it's something really special. From underwear or pants. I just throw the offending clothes away. During one bad change I even threw away the changing pad cover. No thanks. No desire to clean that up.

My kids tag team me now. I can see my son whisper instruction to his little sister. Plotting against me. They scatter in different directions for the second they are out of my control in public. There hits a point where if you have kids like mine, you feel like it's constant and that the only break you get is when they are asleep. Your kids are not going to want to leave the park when it's time to go. Fits will be pitched. Your kids aren't going to want to sit down and behave at the restaurant. They will scream and thro things and ruin other people's meals. Your kids will pull items off the shelves at the grocery store. Chaos follows and ensues everywhere you go.

I've found that tolerance and patience are available in very finite quantities proportional to:

1) your caffeine levels
2) amount of sleep
3) simultaneous crisis
4) love and appreciation for your situation.

When I grant my children additional patience and tolerance I have to take it from somewhere else, usually other adults I encounter. While parenthood has mellowed me as they say, it's made me refocus and I ignore most of what goes on around me, with a few exceptions. I have no patience for idiot adults who want to waste my time. I want everything that doesn't relate to my children to be done as quickly as possible in as short a steps as possible. I was on a webinar the other day and it just could not get to the point and I found myself so intolerant of the time suckage that I stayed signed on but walked away to attend to my children. I watched the Amazing Spiderman and Friends instead of a work related PowerPoint and felt pretty damn good about my decision.

I find myself cleaning the same 3 foot radius in my kitchen over and over and over and over and over again, every day, every week. Holy smokes my neck and shoulders and getting tense just thinking about it. I clean the floor and counter 8-10 times a day. Same spot. Same kids. Same spills. Is it me not learning my lessons? There are days where I spend all day either making food, cleaning up after food and kids and dogs and going from stain to stain to accident to spill then the normal dishes, laundry, bathrooms to then arguing with my children at every turn, with every diaper change, clothing change for every errant behavior. It's exhausting and it's the one thing that really makes me feel like a bad parent when I spend all day feeling pissed off and pissy and like I didn't have one positive moment or interaction with my kids. Where everything was nagging angry mom who was resentful of her role and not good loving and supportive to her children. How am I supposed to work on the big picture items and tackle the learning and more advanced development when I'm drowning in the quagmire of poop and pee and feeding and making sure they are dressed and their teeth are brushed? It's a hard job. It's a hard ass job. One of the tenants of parenting I'm finding is that the feeling that you are making progress or moving forward to very difficult to come by. Because you are doing the same tasks, feeding, cleaning, changing, bathing, snacking, walking, over and over and over again it rarely seems as if things are moving in a forward direction. You are in an overwhelming quagmire of jackassary and sameness.

39. How To Still Be YOU And Be A Parent.

The other mothers I encounter, these bitches don't swear. They say please to their kids all of the time. Please don't set the house on fire. Please don't punch mommy in the face. I'm at war with my kids. I've got Mohmar Khadafi over here, wearing me down, utilizing guerrilla tactics to break my spirit or at the very least my concentration so they can wreak havoc. Now that I have 2 kids, I see them. I see them off in a corner plotting against me. Waiting until I leave the room to push the barstools over to the counter so they can get up and grab scissors and drugs from the cabinets. There is more of them than there are of us now and they are strong and loud and powerful and don't know any fear or boundaries. I don't want to be the nice lady at the park when their kid is having a melt down and throwing sand and being an absolute hulk terror monster saying 'now son please settle down or you are going to get a time out.' I want to whap my kid in the head and tell him to knock it off, with expletives. But I can't. What will the other moms think of me. Just the other day while walking my kids, my 3 year old who is now big enough to walk with me most of the time instead of riding in the double stroller, starting running through a newly landscaped front yard. Here in California everyone is replacing their grass with rocks, and it looks awful BTW, but the kids think its super fun and want to run in it and displace all of the rocks. Uggghh. So my son is running through the rocks clearly in the neighbors yard and I start yelling at him. He won't listen so I grab him by the arm to get him out of their yard and try to get him in the stroller. He's fighting with me tooth and nail. I whap him on the head. Not concussion strength but definitely "I'm serious snap out of it" velocity. A neighbor is driving by. He sees part of this and stops and is staring at me. F U buddy. Its my kid and if I want to try and wrangle him with physical force instead of saying please that is still my prerogative. I felt very guilty about it. I do man handle my kids sometimes. I'm old and tired and if I don't want to wait for them to do something I pick them up and move them along. If they aren't compliant I grab them and take them out of a situation or put them in a stroller and make them wear seatbelts which the older one just hates. It's punishment. I'm sure there are a million different techniques and I'm sure there is something more effective and violence begets violence and all of that but when my daughter undoes the child proof locks and pulls out something dangerous from the cabinets I will smack her hand every time. Even Caesar Milan gives 'corrections' for dogs to snap them out of bad behavior and let them know you are serious. It's a tough one. There are so many challenges trying to get your child in line. I have good ones too. I have wonderful children. They aren't cream puffs. They are tough. And they need to be to be successful in this world. I do believe that much. But they aren't all sweet and kind. They are difficult to control from time to time but who and what isn't. I don't get it right. Not by a long shot. I'm too short tempered and quick to yell. But I also don't believe in saying please don't hit me. Say it enough and it's meaningless. My kid punches me I'm going to get their attention so they know at least for that moment not to do it again. Do you smack, punch, pinch, what? Spanking through diapers is absolutely worthless and it hurts your hand more than it hurts them. I try holding their arms down, their legs down, push on them to get them to sit in a car seat so I can buckle them in when they are arching their backs and kicking and screaming, and of course people are watching me and getting their phones out to call CPS on me.

Raising your kids is kind of like the "Dog Whisperer." You need to walk them. You need to wear them out. You need to be the leader, the alpha dog. You need to break their attention when they are misbehaving and try to redirect them. Having been a step parent for years I realized early that to be the leader I had to act like the leader. Be in charge. Be the parent, not always the friend, but the stable and ever present authority in their lives. I tell new parents that the hard part feels like those first few months, but really it's when they start walking. Once your child becomes mobile the real work begins. It's like that Swifter commercial, once they are mobile and motoring around there is no deep couch sitting. You are always on the edge of grabbing your child, and try grabbing their shirt instead of their arm all of the time. I put marks on my kids arms from grabbing them and trying to avert disaster 100 times a day by catching them in the nick of time. My husband once grabbed my son who had somehow used a storage container as a step stool and then monkey feet climbed up onto the counter and was trying to walk around and fell off. He got him by the pants and it was like Tom Cruise in Mission Impossible dangling mere inches from crashing head first on the tile floor. It's constant, and even when you figure out how to contain them, there are a MILLION things they can still hurt themselves on and trouble they can get into. They have a sixth sense, if there is something new in the environment that is potentially dangerous or deadly they will be there faster than you can ever imagine. It will scare you. You are tired. You will be caught off guard at how fast a mobile child can get into a world of hurt.

These ladies I run into over and over again all seem to have the same script, the same cantor to their voices. That mom voice that is sweet and polite and please and thank you. They are like telemarketers that all have gotten the same script and you are trying to talk to them with logic and reason and they can't go off the script. It's maddening. Plus I'm not like that so I feel judged. Constantly judged. The joke however is on them because I know they are secretly jealous of how confident I am, though they judge my kids cleanliness and manners, but jealous of how self assured I seem in the face of infinite choices and no clear direction. One thing I can tell you is that sometimes the soft approach does work. Lowering your voice so they have to listen good to hear you instead of yelling and gently moving them along instead of grabbing them or picking them up. But damn, that is a lot of work and I'm so tired and borderline embarrassed and constantly apologizing in public and none of the techniques will really stop a true meltdown, the only thing that works is taking your kid out of the situation and dealing with it privately, in your car if you are out or in your home. I'm not Mrs. Cleaver, not by a long shot, but even with all of my mistakes my kids still love me and every once in a while an older person will give me a nod of approval when I'm not all sunshine and polite when my kids are absolute asshole terrors. I'm Rick Ross. I'm the boss.

40. Unsolicited Advice. The Scourge Of New Mom Existence.

I have very educated, smart and outspoken friends who have offered a litany of advice over the past few years. From how to get pregnant, to the amount of food and exercise to have, and all of the bases of raising a child. How often and when to have sex to conceive was some sage advice from a dear friend. Her point was that the vitality and effectiveness of sperm delivery dissipated if you have sex every day. She said every other day for 3 days around ovulation. BTW conceiving my last baby we had sex for 5 days in a row with my estimated ovulation date in the middle of that. She also said to potty train her kids right away. Which she did. She had her 2 boys that are a year apart fully trained at almost 3 and almost 2. She had a plastic urinal in their bathroom. Wow. She also has 2 nannies and the kids started school immediately. I dragged my heels training my son, and at 3 ½ he still wasn't trained. I felt it as a badge of honor instead of something to be ashamed of. What it meant to me was I was privileged that my kid wasn't in daycare fulltime and didn't have other people in charge of his day, yet. Is it a pain in the ass to have an almost 40 pound 3 ½ foot tall three year old in diapers. Yes. He's hard to lift and he hasn't fit on my changing table for quite a while. Oh well. I've made things harder on myself but I watch my friends and peers train their boys very early and its just rough because there is a self awareness component that is missing. My son knows when he's wet and when he has to poop and quite frankly its easier to change 2 sets of diapers every few hours then sitting on top of my son every 15 minutes to monitor if he needs to go.

The hardest part about unsolicited advice is to not take it in as a criticism and to start defending yourself, as I did in the above paragraph. I always saw it was you are doing this wrong let me tell you how to do it right. Its difficult to reconcile that and to turn it around to see that its merely someone's opinion and maybe something that worked for them that may or may not work for you. Really then it should always start with, "I'd love to help you by telling you this tip or technique that helped me." Never does though. Through judgy eyes and a stepped in dog poop pinched face you have someone, usually a woman, I'm just saying, tell you something about what you should be doing instead of what you are currently doing. Then you start defending yourself with 'well at home we do this but I'm out in public.' Uggghhh.

Some advice that haunts me, even today, because it was solid and I didn't heed it. I didn't even think about taking it. I actually got a little mad when I got it like give me a break why are you telling me this what do you think I'm stupid. I am stupid. It's hard to discern who is just nosy putting in their 2 cents and getting advice you can actually use. These words echo in my head today:

"I wish I had laid off the ice cream a bit. If I had kept just an extra 10 pounds off during pregnancy I'd be so much happier now." Advice given during a lunch meeting with a friend who had a 6 month old while I was pregnant with my son. She was still wearing maternity jeans because her pre pregnancy pants didn't fit. I lost all but 10 pounds I gained while pregnant with my son by the time he was 8 months old. I was back in hot mamma jeans that I liked. My daughter was a whole other story. I got so stuck trying to get even a pound off. She's over 1 at this point and I'm still 20+ pounds away from where I want to be and I work my ass off 5 days a week and lose all of the ground by relaxing the other 2. It's a complete battle and while I don't regret for a second any meals I ate while pregnant I really don't remember them and if I had maybe kept a cap on the excessive sweets and snacks vs. meals I would be in a different scenario. I was very childish and cavalier about my eating and weight gain while pregnant. I should learn a lesson from it because the over indulgence laid the groundwork for how I eat on a regular basis and it became the habit, the norm, instead of a treat.

"Don't let them in your bed. Once they get in you will never get them out." Advice given to me by 3 sources but the exact quote came from one of the nurses who took care of me post delivery after my son was born. I didn't listen. He's was my baby and at the time I thought he might be my only one and if I want to sleep with him that's my choice. He slept with me almost every nap and night until he was 6 months old then I tried to get him in a crib. Oh my god the howling, the crying. I waited the recommended 20 minutes to see if he would drift off to sleep. Oy vey that didn't work and I got so worried about him burning off the precious breast feeding calories by crying his eyes out that I caved. I got him there though. Right around 8 months I had him in his crib for naps and at night for most of the time for a full week. Then he got a slight cold and we had an emotional crisis and he was right back in. That's where parenting kicks your ass because the mistakes are made when you are down and distracted and crazed. I let up on the gas for a second, a few nights, and that was it. It became easier to have him sleep with me then dealing with the nonsense and tantrums and crying and energy involved in putting him down in his own room. I didn't get him out again until he was 3 ½ and I had to buy him a zippy sack and put his bed in our room. He still comes in with me from time to time but he's much more independent.

My little girl, 2nd baby, was all bassinet for the first few weeks then crib. I learned my lesson. I even kicked all of the dogs out of my bed. My sleep is more important than almost anything in the house, well not really but it's on the list and I've had too many sleepless nights where I'm being kicked and punched and moved off my own bed. Put on your oxygen mask before you put on your child's. Wish I had listened. Learned my lesson the 2nd time around. Mostly. Actually not all of the time. My family is Mexican so we all sleep together sometimes but joking aside with some emotional set backs over the last few years we are lost unless we all sleep together. It's a sacrifice but we are good making it for now. We did kick the dogs out, well most of them and during most of the night, so that's progress.

"Watch what you eat after you stop nursing and aren't burning those extra 500 calories a day." Well that pretty much sums it up. I have taste buds to satisfy. Life at a stay at home mom is structured but not in a sense that you have access to your refrigerator and pantry all day. When you go to work you bring or buy food and you usually have a finite amount and limited access due to supply or time. At home not so much. It's always there and if you are like me you are always feeding kids. With 2 little ones I find I move from diaper to snack to diaper to drink to snack to meal to diaper to snack to meal to dessert. I also like to make all of my kids happy and I'm not very regimented about what they eat. I look at their food consumption on a continuum. Over the course of a few days or even a week to find a good balance. I feel its almost impossible during the course of a single day to have a perfect balance of fruit, veggies, lean proteins, good fats, carbs, water, milk, juice and treats. So we have junk food, we have kid food, and there are days when my kids are choosing apples as I'm eating the last of the Oreos. Damn you cookies, why you have to taste so good? WHY!?!

"My Kid is ...walking, talking, reading, writing, working for NASA already ... how about yours" I'm a pretty confident person. I don't waiver to much once I make a decision, I don't second guess myself often but I found myself back on my heels so many times during the first few years of my son's life. I actually doubted myself. I was overwhelmed by peer pressure, not even pressure but feeling jealous and competitive. One of my best friend has uber kids. Touched by the hand of God. Came out big and healthy and she had them potty trained immediately and in academy and reading and writing before they were 3 and trips and vacation and just super kids. She is an amazing business woman and her husband is a former USC Quarterback. Their kids are big, smart, athletic, were potty trained by 2 and started school around the same time. For their 4th and 5th birthdays they started their own charity that they sit on the board meetings of and help organize fundraising events. Hard to keep up with that. I felt like that scene from Parenthood where the brother-in-law says 'Patty is learning the Piano' or something, and Steve Martin's character says, 'is Patty a doctor yet?' Cut to his kid wearing a bucket on his head and ramming into the wall and eating stickers. That's how I felt. If I only knew. I feel like I was too insecure and made some stupid decisions out of that fear of not being on track. Plus kids are like animals. They smell fear. I started feeding my kid anything he would eat because I was afraid he was under weight. I let my kid sleep where ever he want because I felt like he didn't sleep enough. I watched other people in our immediate circle and what I saw was insanely polite, compliant, calm kids and I felt like I had the anti Christ. I do not. My son is sweet and loving and generous and a little boy. He is awesome and my flaw as a parent is when I try to keep up with everyone else or get back on my heels with all of the inquiries about what achievements he has and where he is at school and I get defensive and start yelling at him for things that are just him being a kid. Not just a kid but MY kid with my personality traits and following the path I've laid out for him. He is absolutely amazing and I love him so much. I saw their best and compared it to my worst. Ugggh. I blame it on the lack of sleep. I blame it on ignorance. I didn't know it was ok and it was all going to even out.

I ran into a local mom at the park who just told me about her child's diagnosis of being on the "autism spectrum." The kid started talking late. She is his first. The kid is fine and has no problems from what I have seen but he started talking late so now he has this anti social non verbal diagnosis. The mom in response treats him a little like something is wrong with him, so do the other kids that interact with him on a regular basis. She's nervous so he's nervous so everyone is nervous. Now everyone at the park knows he doesn't like to be chased or have people make loud noises around him, so of course the other kids chase him around and make loud noises. Sometimes you fit your kid into that diagnosis though, it's sitting in your consciousness that something is wrong so you treat your child like something is wrong until eventually something is wrong. I do my best in those situation to say something flippant which I'm sure some would consider rude but I told her straight out, your kid is fine. Nothing wrong with him. I've looked him in the eyes. I've engaged with him. If he is having problems they are slight and shouldn't be ruling his life like they are. My kids eats cardboard and likes to drink lotion and shampoo. Some call this Pica, I call it him being an idiot and maybe I didn't nurse him long enough and I never got him on a pacifier but I sucked my thumb for like forever so it's just a biting, eating, oral things and if he eats and subsequently poops out a few plastic dinosaurs we will live and the last thing I want to do is take him in and have him diagnosed as having a problem. It's the road to ruin. Some kids are slower than others. That's the way it goes. Their milestone time line speaks nothing of their hearts, or their souls, or who they are as people, just which tasks they have either picked up or have shoved down their throats until they started repeating them.

"They need to be in school right away to get them socialized. What classes and activities are they in?" It's soapbox time. My sister is a PhD. She went to school until she was 30. There is enough school in their future for me. I want them to have no schedule right now, be free, explore, learn, create, be themselves. Organic is my code word for I'm being lazy but I'm not. It's my privilege and my gift right now to be a stay at home mom with no strict schedule. We don't have to be up or anywhere at any given time. We got to parks and for walks and play and have a blast each and every day. I'm glad to feed and change and dress them. It's my honor. I'm sure they could care it's me doing all of the small duties but I also don't feel good about paying someone else to do it either. No one will watch my kid the way I do. Period. I change diapers immediately. No one walks around poopie or hungry at my house.

No I don't have a strict schedule and fill our days with dozens of activities. Outdoor and playtime are number one to me. We are trying art classes and music classes and sports. My husband says it well let the 'kids be kids' as long as possible. They want ice cream? Sure. They want to sleep in? Let them have at it as life will catch up at some point and they will be on a strict schedule. Let them be happy and kids as long as they can.

Guess what? I'm SO GUILTY of giving ridiculous advice and putting in my two cents. I do it so much more than I even realize. I am the problem.

41. And Now MY 2 Cents On Some Hot Button Topics Aka Some Unsolicited Advice.

My opinion is worth what you paid for it right? Here is my stance on a few issues. Keeping in mind that I have been pregnant 3 times in 5 years, going from being a full time executive to a stay at home mom, that I've had high risk pregnancies and all of the doctoring that goes into that and that I have a lot of strong women in my life that love to share their wisdom which is code for nag me to death and make me feel like I'm doing something wrong and finally that I am confident enough to be able to differentiate between people I believe and trust and those who I think are full of crap as well as seek out help and advice when I truly need and want it.

Baby Brain. Yes it's real. I think it is a combination of exhaustion, hormones and distraction. You are exhausted but eventually your body adjusts to the lack of sleep, the interrupted sleep patterns, lack of REM, having to be on ultra high alert while you are sleeping and all of that. It takes a while but you start feeling ok even and get used to it. You also have a bunch of hormones surging through your system. Pregnancy hormones, post pregnancy hormones, breastfeeding hormones if you went that route, and the addition of birth control hormones and in my case pre-menopausal hormones. It's a mess. Finally you are distracted. There is someone in your field of vision, your ear shot, your mind space who is infinitely more important than you and needs the most careful and detailed care you can give. Given this perfect storm of factors I can tell you that my short term memory is gone and my long term recall is seriously warped. Baby brain is a giant fog, that you struggle and squint to see through and you are moving through your actions and your day and you don't feel like anything is stable or clear. You find yourself mentally grasping for a fact or a name that was right there only a few moments ago and now it's gone. You find yourself mentally stuttering, trying to make or worse get out a thought. It's that frustration of walking upstairs to get something only to forget why you went there in the first place then get distracted by something else. It's calling your kid by your dog's name and putting your nice china in the trash and a paper plate in the sink.

The silver lining is that its slowly coming back with sleep and use. The more I play jeopardy at night the better I play the next day which is all about my long term recall. The more uninterrupted sleep I get the better my short term processes. I'm not sure if I'll ever be back where I was but that's fine by me because what I have now is actually better. What I have now is the notion, the philosophy, the reality that I have bigger fish to fry so I am extremely effective and efficient and I don't mess around in my actions or my thinking. I want to knock that problem out so I can be with my kids. Gravity Falls is on in 10 minutes and I have a ton to get done so I'm going to wizard my skills and get it all done so I can hang out with my husband and my kids. So when your brain does start firing again, it's genius. Your brain has been sitting in recoil position, building up energy and momentum. When you can make something happen or have a good focused thought, as Mr. Jay would say on America's Next Top Model, "It's genius."

Self Confidence. Are you kidding. I'm old and fat and have 2 kids but I feel close to the best I've ever felt. I survived high risk pregnancies, I have amazing children, I survived child birth and my body and brain have seen better days but damn if I don't feel invincible and as long as my husband still wants to have sex with me it's I'm happy. While I was pregnant with my son, which was plagued with more mental and emotional stress than I would ever wish on anyone, I felt like a frickin' superhero. My body felt amazing. I feel close to that. I don't feel much doubt about anything anymore. Not only did I get through all of the trials and tribulations of the last few years, I've come out better and stronger and I'm really to kick some ass. Being a parent doesn't give you the luxury of being wishy washy, of being a wuss, of being shy, of being a wall flower, of being indecisive. Time to shine your light on the world, on yourself and to set an example for your kids.

Justifying myself to the world
I do feel defensive of my position and for some reason compelled to sneak in the information that I did not have IVF. I want people to know it was all natural, God's work, no medical intervention. Just good old fashioned sex and then a baby. Unless prenatal vitamins count towards enhancing my chances the only preparation I did was clean up my lifestyle a bit. I was a smoker. For some reason I had this thought that I'd quit when I got pregnant. I didn't really drink but I smoked and occasionally smoked weed. All that had to go by the wayside to get pregnant. But I did not harvest my eggs, I did not have my child in a lab then have the embryo reinserted. I feel for anyone who has to undergo that type of intervention but seriously if you want a baby and that's your option it's not a bad option at all. In fact it's pretty effective if you think about it. I had to rely on my husband having sex with me at the right time, a time I had to calculate and of course after I actually started getting hard core about calculating that with my third and last pregnancy I became more and more unsure about when that actual date was. I must have lucked out and hit it the first two times. I want to tell people with my first 2 pregnancies we really only tried once. Once. One 10 minute act of sex during the entire few weeks up to and after the actual conception. Just once. But it makes me sound borderline undesirable and my husband like he isn't doing his job at our house. So I have to justify myself in another way here. I have one of the best marriages I know how. I'm so stupidly happy I just glow all of the time and the worry and anxiety of my previous life has passed into the distance. Everything however is a compromise and I compromised having a lot of sex for having a lot of happiness. My husband's cousin is a few months older than me and her son is a year older than ours. She and I see eye to eye on the first few years as she is a long time stay at home mom. If your kid is already smart and athletic and all of that all they need is encouragement but going to a certain school wont' make them intrinsically smarter or going to a boat of sports clinics and camps and leagues won't make them more athletic. Hard work and encouragement are vital to the development of any talent but you can't change what you were given. You can improve upon it with a lot of work but you either have it or you don't. I am constantly

bombarded with inquiries about my son's schooling and sports teams and learning curriculum and we have none. I'm winging it and doing my best to provide what I think is a happy loving fun home. I'm not worried about his development one iota but I find myself sometimes occupied with doubt. Am I doing him a disservice by keeping him with me? Hurting him to make myself feel happy and content. Being a stay at home mom is so underrated. You are the mom, the lady with the bat shit crazy kids who is yelling at them and making a scene at the grocery store.

42. Fidgety Parents. It's Torture.

Lord help me. I guess being old takes some of the neurosis out of child rearing. I'm very relaxed about a lot of things because I'm too tired to fight them and I really weigh how important they are to me and the big picture. Not all of the parents I encounter take this road however. There is an uptight range that I admire for having a philosophy and sticking to their rules but come on. There are the food Nazi moms. I've encountered quite a few. I strive to balance my children's diets. I also try to look at food on a continuum. While one meal might not be the best; i.e. a box of Willy Wonka nerds, a PowerAde, and some tortilla chips, I look at everything they eat over the course of a few days or even a week to make sure I get in their fresh fruit, vegetables and good proteins. I don't stress if they eat treats before meals, as I find that taking the taboo out of that concept actually guides them towards making better choices. But I digress. One nut job I ran into at a Superbowl party blew me away. My son is a love He can be rough from time to time but for the most part a very generous loving child. He was a few months shy of his 3rd birthday and I was pregnant. He made a friend of a little 4 year old girl at this party. He went to a small table in the television area and grabbed two cookies. One for him and one for his friend. As he went to hand the cookie to his new friend here comes monster mom. "Oh no. She can't have that. I don't let her have sugar." Really no sugar I say. That must be difficult. "Yes I really have to stay on top of it and monitor everything she eats and read labels diligently." Good for you. That's too much work for me and good luck with that. For anyone who thinks they have a good bead on everything their kids eat, your parents, your partner, your husbands, your children's siblings have already given them something off of your taboo list, and that's a fact. Along with the household cleaners, dog hair and the occasional bug they have ingested foods that you do not approve of. Sorry to burst your bubble.

Another mom I've had the privilege of indirectly dealing with has her child on a holistic macrobiotic diet. I know the grandparents. Who make a point since they think the child is malnourished, thin and are always on the border of calling CPS, to feed the child a mess of junk food every time they take care of her. Pizza, hot dogs, candy, ice cream. The child then becomes monstrously sick after their visits. Nice. Excellent grand parenting. BTW not all grandparents are good grandparents. Some of them really suck at it and just because they are older and had kids themselves doesn't make them an expert, or hell even competent

Now I get it. Your child is precious. You want to control any harmful influences from getting around them. I feel the same way. I guess I'm just to tired and lazy to be as strict. We go to the park all of the time. The toddler focused parks in our neighborhood have sand and the ones for the older kids have bark. We run into tons of different groups of moms and dads and kids. It never fails. One of the ladies I know from the area has a one year old. Same age as my daughter. When my 3 year old gets near her child at the park she freaks out. He's going to get him dirty. He's going to get sand in his eyes. She comments that my son is too rough. My kid is sweet. He does throw sand from time to time, never intentionally on someone, well hardly ever. Keep in mind we are in a park that is filled with a few metric tons of sand so yes sand does fly from time to time. The weird part is this woman really wants to talk to me, she can see me on my walking route through the neighborhood from her backyard and ends up meeting up with me at the park when I'm done. But then she freaks out when my kids are next to hers. I don't get it. I do but I don't. Parenting becomes about your ego. What your tolerance levels are. I feel like I'm trying to let my children explore boundaries. Am I just being a lazy parent who isn't my child enough discipline?

The next level of parenting I find myself faced with is the overly ambitious parents who are constantly pushing their children. How about an insane list of activities, and no a 3 year old shouldn't need a day planner to coordinate and track their schedules, and if they do it's overload already. The Dance Mom parents who made it a competition as the baby was pushing out of the womb. From the inane bragging about statistics, to their placement on the growth charts, this is just the beginning of the never ending race of meaningless statistics and anxiety over whether or not their kid is bigger than yours. Next I'm sure will be kindergarten spelling tests and how many goals the kids had at soccer. So nip your stress over it in the bud and take it all with a grain of salt. Most of the numbers are meaningless and truthfully the only person concerned about your child's place on a growth chart is you and your pediatrician. The only one who cares how many goals your child scored is your husband, so he can brag about it to his friends.

The key I've found to managing parents who are trying a little too hard, and are too focused on relaying all of the braggadocios information about their offspring is the following:
"That is amazing. You must be so proud." Or something very similar. What they are looking for really is your praise that their child and therefore the parents are exceptional and special. It does not hurt you for a minute to see when someone is really aiming to let you know how wonderful their kid is to let them know that yes their child is amazing. You don't need to go tit for tat and start spewing statistics back. Acknowledge, praise, and move on.

43. Mind Set Of Being A LIL (Late In Life) Mon And Dealing With Ancient Grandparents.

There are a lot of realities that will set in for the older mom. On the plus side, you are more confident, and or too tired to give a crap and get caught up in the neurotic insecurities of the peer group game. I am not doing what the moms around me are with regards to preschool and athletics. Sorry but basketball at 3 is ridiculous. Most moms I encounter have their kids in all day preschool (or daycare as its more commonly called) because everyone else does. They start soccer at 3 because everyone else does. Martial arts because everyone else does. While I feel the anxiety from time to time when everyone else around me is doing the same thing and I'm not part of that group, I sit back and think I'm making my choices for my children and not succumbing to group think and they're going to be just fine.

Along the same lines, being older I have a better outlook on paths, strategies, potential outcomes. I was able to buy a house, before I had kids, in an amazing family orientated neighborhood with a blue ribbon award winning elementary school. There will be no second guessing or scrambling to get my kids in a good school or even a commute. We are set for the next 10 years walking our children to one of the best schools in the state. Foresight. Planning. Financial savvy. Some of the perks of being older. Living off of prior investments. I haven't worked for a steady paycheck in over 4 years. I'm putting my brain power to use to redefine a career that allows me to be with my kids during these precious first years.

Another hard fact is that your children may have a very limited relationship with their grandparents, if any at all. My mom had me when she was 20 so I had 2 full sets of grandparents and even a great grandmother and great aunts. My kids don't have that. My parents are in their late 60's and early 70's and my husband's mom passed away before our kids were born and my father in law is in his mid 70's. Now the notion that if our kids waited as long as we did to have children we may not live to be grandparents ourselves. You may never get to experience the joy of being a grandparent, of helping your children raise their children. To be there when you children are adults to guide them and offer a shoulder to lean on. Our time with our children is going to be more greatly limited than our parents time was with us. That one stings and I find myself writing letters to all of my children with everything from how to do something to how to feel about themselves, just in case I'm not around to tell them in person.

44. Wrap it up!

Here is what I'm left with aside from the two most important most loved miracles of my life and I can't remember anything before. I love my kids so much it makes my cry when I stare at them and think about how I almost missed it all. How I didn't know and I didn't care and I wasn't moving my life in a direction that was going to get me here. I wasn't looking for a partner and I wasn't taking care of myself well enough to land one if I stumbled across one. How lucky I am. How blessed.

From a dressed in all black LA girl to wearing as much vivid color as possible, all Oprah-esque I LOVE COLOR!!! Living single for so long and trying to be hip and cool and failing miserably I almost always dressed in black and surrounded myself w black and white and gray. The vibrant colors kids bring into your world is a total mood booster. Forget that smoothie just be around a bunch of crazy hued kiddie toys and that will put a smile on your face. After my daughter I found myself wanting to wear color all of the time. To reflect the happiness and joy and to be uplifting and upbeat and also it helps that when you dress in bright colors it makes it easier for the kids to find you. Love bright colors at public places like the park and the zoo. I can find them and they can find me. I also now agree w dressing the kids in the same shirts so they can find each other and you can see them easier. Being a mom especially of more than one requires special force level tactics and honing your senses. My eye sight is impaired by so many factors including total lack of sleep, lack of quality sleep, post pregnancy on set allergies, pregnancy and post pregnancy changes in my vision, old age catching up skewing my eyesight and eye dryness and last but not least getting regularly punched and poked and squirted in the eye. Children have no regard for the sanctity of vision. They think eyes are fun to poke and hit and throw things at. So much fun.

Now I know what pregnancy feels like. What labor feels like and it's so unbelievably cool to have those memories. I'll admit that I've taken about ½ a dozen pregnancy tests since my last baby and even at the 6 week post delivery check up when I had my Mirena birth control implant installed I was worried I was pregnant.

Those symptoms are pretty distinct. Not a few weeks ago my back was killing me, like back labor. My stomach and digestive systems were a mess, like they were at the tail end of my pregnancy, and my boobs hurt as did my joints, and I was getting headaches and weird food cravings and no matter how hard I worked out I couldn't make the scale budge. All to me indicators of pregnancy and I kept having moments that felt very "I Didn't Know I Was Pregnant" type situation because I really don't get a period anymore, just mild bleeding or spotting and I'm so consumed with my kids that while I'm in touch with my body, ehhh not really and maybe if I had one of those surprise pregnancies I wouldn't have noticed. Unfortunately I think I had food poisoning coupled with the onset of menopause, but dammit it's fun to dream sometimes and I miss being pregnant and having a little little baby everyday and I do wish I could do it again. I loved it and I'm so so happy and satisfied that I got to experience it.

No one gets away clean here. I am a very self assured person. Something about having kids. The enormity and importance of having someone else's life in your hands. The responsibility of doing everything you can to make your kids safe, healthy, nice, educated, and all of that. The daily struggle of did I feed them good and healthy foods and enough of it, to are we putting good habits and information into them for the future. I forgot to feed my son lunch once. Lunch. Oh I ate, I don't miss any meals but I forgot to feed him lunch. What is wrong with me. Exhaustion leads to self doubt. Feeling overwhelmed leads to self doubt. In my case being older and very tired and arrogant but not having been around of lot of people who have kids because I was older and when my friends started having kids they faded away because I didn't. Who wants to be that creepy friend at the kids birthday parties who doesn't have a kid.

I found that the majority of my parenting decisions on a day to day in the trenches basis revolve around how loud my child is screaming. I make terrible decisions all to get him or her to just be quiet and stop screeching or crying or yelling. I want to trade anything, I mean anything to stop their unhappiness. A 4th Otter

Pop, at 10 o clock at night, absolutely if you will just stop crying. I'm in the middle of having 5 minutes to try and work out but you won't stop having a complete melt down unless I stop and pick you up, you got it kid. It's like eating a donut after dieting all day. I feel that all of the caving I do just to get them to stop screaming erases all of the other work I do and all of the will power I exercise and the parental power and control and good decisions I make during the day are gone. Parenting is in the moment. It's crisis management. Do I let my kid be unhappy and cry and scream? I tried that for sleep training with my son. I had him with me as an infant so I could nurse and he never took to the bassinet plus I didn't know if I would ever have the experience again so I had him sleep with me, on top of me, right next to me. I love it. Well so did he because when I finally tried to crib train him, OMG what a nightmare. Let him cry for 20 minutes I would read or see on TV. Let him be in distress. Then I would panic about his calories, what if he burns so many calories it erases all of the nursing I managed to get in during the day. I worked at getting him crib trained. I unplugged the monitors and let him cry. I will tell you he NEVER fell asleep that way. EVER. The most I let him go was 40 minutes and to this day I regret all of it. My child is fine now. He will sleep anywhere. He will sleep when he's tired. There is something about making them or letting them be so distressed that I feel works the opposite and fuels their fire and just creates a whole mess of unhappiness for everyone. At the end of the day I want happy, loved kids and a decent environment. Maybe that is the kicker about being older. The alleged maturity and ability to see longer term horizons while in the thick of it all.

BTW your kids have super crappy judgment. While they might be pissed off and unhappy in the moment and they want it now, and it's not going to kill them to wait a few minutes. HOWEVER trust me on this, they WILL MAKE YOU PAY. Everyday I find when I take that extra few minutes to take care of myself, or clean, or even trying to write this book, and I let them fuss or be disgruntled even in a total controlled environment, they will find a way to do something so messy or destructive that it makes you wish you had taken that extra 2-3 minutes to make them happy or appease them because the result is 10-20 minutes of clean up or frustration or suffering on your part to fix it afterwards.

Parenting is managing ever present layers of insecurity on a moment by moment basis while trying to maintain some working level of your long term goals for how you want to behave and how you want your child to behave and how you want to shape their environment and judgment and reactions. It's a nearly impossible task, especially when tired and stressed. The world isn't going to cooperate. Your child certainly isn't going to cooperate, so how do you persist. This is the largest part of my daily struggle. All of the while I'm telling myself I'm smart why can't I manage all of this better or more effectively or make it all go much much much smoother. There are days where I truly do just want to give up. I'll let my kids cry way longer than I ordinarily would. I let those wet diapers stay on far too long. I lay down and just let them rip the upstairs apart and quietly hope and pray that they don't hurt themselves. I'll deal with the mess and all of that later. I get tired of the fight. The fight to get dressed, to eat, to bathe, to change their diaper. I give up. They will eat when they are hungry and sleep when they are tired.

This is a great way to wrap this all up because we all feel the same way. None of us do a perfect job, and those that think they do are way off. Righteousness and justification come with the job. Some parents are better than others. That's the way it goes. Some are born with it. Some learn it. Some are so dedicated they can't not fail.

I have and know true JOY. Cliché to the core. I'll say what every other parent will tell you. Nothing in life was ever as important as my kids are now. Nothing mattered and maybe it's the lack of sleep and inability to focus with kids yelling in my ear and the smell of pee overwhelming my nose and someone always crawling all over me numbing my sense of feel but I don't remember life before kids. The impact and the joy is so significant and so intense it is like nothing I had ever experienced and even with the hardships and issues we were forced to face on many fronts having children it was worth every single second and I would not go back and do it different. I love and cherish my husband to the millionth degree especially when I watch him being a father, and a top notch kick ass one at that. I am absolutely over the moon rainbows shooting out of my ass madly deeply in love and absolute devoted adoration with my children. Smiles and heart filled with joy when they kiss me or even the oohs and aahs when the do something cool or sweet and the cherry on top of the sundae is in those hidden moments that no one sees but you and they are sweet with each other. All worth it.

V: Buying Guide

45. What Do You Really Need To Bring Baby Home? And My 2 Cents On Baby Items.

Shop 'till you drop on your phone and have a blast with it. Put all kinds of crazy nonsense in your registry, you can always take it out later. But please do make sure you take it out. With multiple registries sometimes you can forget and in my case someone actually bought me one of my outrageous dream items. Ooops. It's fun to dream and to wish. You have this event coming and unlike most of life you know exactly when this one is happening. Planning and preparation can be fun, frivolous, fantastic things to keep your mind off of the impending terror of actually going into labor and giving birth.

The Essentials:

1) Boobs. If you are nursing there is your food supply. And it's pretty much free. Cha Ching. **$0**

2) Diapers. Hear me on this one. There are differences in quality and effectiveness with different diaper brands. Diapers can be a hard expense to add to your shopping line up. A box of diapers from the Costco runs about $40-50 and will last you 3-4 weeks depending on how often you change them. Here is my brand run down. Kirkland/Costco brand is just fine. I used them time and time again with very little leaking on a boy or a girl. My kids didn't blow their diapers out much. I change my kids as soon as they are muddy or wet whenever possible. I found the Costco brand to be a good value and a good brand. Also Pampers and Huggies that have the elastic type waist in the back and elastic leg openings. Those work really well. Do you best to size your diapers appropriately. Too small doesn't work at all and too big just opens you up to a lot of leaks and messes. As my son is going through his year of potty training I buy Luvs, they are the cheapest diapers and I don't care how well they perform because again I change poo poo's right away and he does his pee pees mostly in the potty at this point. Same with the generic grocery and drug store brands, they aren't very good but effective if you are potty training, etc. I wouldn't use those for babies though. They are cheap and they do leak. Spend the extra $10 for the good quality diapers for the first 2 years. The extra you spend on diapers you will save in time, energy, water, soap, and effort cleaning up messes on your kids clothes and on your furniture and floors. **$25-50**

3) Wipes. After trying several brands and utilizing various coupons I come back to the same brand over and over. Kirkland from Costco. The best wipes on the market at the highest value. They are the most versatile, you can use them on anything but your floors, makes them too slippery because there is a little bit of aloe / lotion in them. They don't have a nasty taste to them and they stay together. I tried to save a few bucks a few weeks ago by using coupons and buying the value pack of a leading brand vs. the Kirkland ones. The other ones came in a few giant bags that you need to store and manage, gotta seal them tight or all few thousand wipes will dry out. Also you have to have good wipe containers to put them in. The Kirkland wipes are self contained and just have a closing access on top of a packet. Easy to deal with and easy to store. I have packs of them all over the house and in the car and in the stroller. The others require the hard boxes and don't taste good and the wipe not only falls apart it is textured which sounds advantageous to get off poop but it actually has been chaffing my poor baby's bottom because it grabs. Kirkland all of the way. Everyday. All day. For babies, for you, for dogs, for the kitchen, for the bathroom, for the car, for your purse, for the stroller. Everywhere and anywhere. Buy them. Don't buy any other ones. Not worth the trouble over a few dollars. **$20**

4) A Few Onesies. Those Gerber white short or long sleeved onesies from the Target for about $12 for a pack of 4-6 are awesome. They have the long sleeved ones with the caps on the ends to cover their little hands so they don't scratch themselves. They are soft and serve their purpose. They also make a front button wrap shirt that is functional and nice. The clothes they wear for that first month are just that. It isn't a fashion show. You aren't going out much. Functional and easy to change is best. You are going to be tired and your fingers are going to fumble over the little snaps. **$10-20**

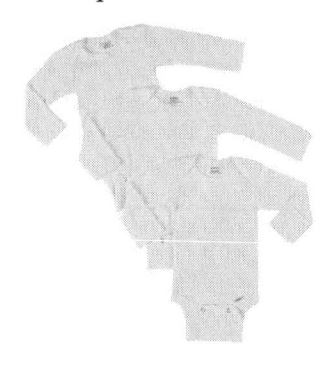

Carters Onesies with Mittens

5) A Place For Baby To Sleep. Bassinet? Crib? Pack n Play? Whatever you want. I had a second hand bassinet and a crib. My wish list was one of those rocking cradles. I didn't make the investment because you can only safely have them sleep in those for a few months. You will find out the hard way that some items they grow out of so fast it wasn't worth it. Having 2 babies in less than 3 years I double used most of my gear and only then did I feel like I got a good value out of it. So I had a repurposed bassinet that I cleaned up well and bought a new mattress for as well a crib with a very nice mattress as well. My kids mostly slept with me. They also sell those Moses baskets for co-sleeping as it's termed. I don't know. You will have to figure it out. If you are nursing having the baby sleep with you is handy. I kept a bassinet at the foot of our bed and a crib in our room until they were older.
$60-600. Basinets about $100, Pack n Play about $75, Cribs start at about $150 plus $100 for a mattress and can go up to $1000 or more.

6) Bottles. Even nursing moms need a few bottles to either feed pre-pumped milk or formula from time to time. I had about 8 for my first kid, 2 for my second. All of the bottles are a little different and you don't know which ones your kids are going to like and want to use ahead of time. You might have to try a few different types to find a good fit. I suggest not buying too many in advance, and buy the smaller packs so you can try a few different brands. **$15-40**

7) *Formula.* I had great luck with the Kirkland by Costco brand for $16 for a huge can. I read the ingredients diligently and also spoke with my doctor about any difference between the 'generic' and the name brands. He didn't see any issues and I didn't see any difference. I used formula to supplement breastfeeding with my first baby so I wasn't too concerned about it and may have made a different decision if I was exclusively using formula. I felt that my baby was getting all of the vitamins and nutrients from me and the formula was truly just a supplement, a sleep aid, and a way for my husband to do some of the feeding and have that bonding experience, well not so much bonding but for me to get some sleep. With formula you need a few bottles and do yourself a favor and spend the $1 and buy the nursery water to mix with versus tap water. I'm not sure if there is any benefit but it makes you feel better. **$16-30/can**

8) *Snot Sucking Bulb Thing.* Cost a few bucks. Worth it if you have a snotty baby. Especially for those first few days there is a lot of fluid etc. that needs to clear out of their little lungs and you will get scared when you hear them choking on their own mucus. Get a few and you will likely get one from the hospital. Grab a few little plastic syringes and dosers as well to help give you baby any medicine or liquid vitamins. **$5**

9) *Boobie Care.* If you are doing the boob thing then at minimum you need to care for your nipples as they are about to take a beating. Generic nipple creams are thick, mostly lanolin. The name brands are thinner. Do you prefer thin or thick lotions, so choose according to your personal preference but you will need it and get in a habit of using it daily. Nursing pads help in a lot of ways, they absorb the extra cream so you don't kill your bras and help with any leaks. The Johnson and Johnson brand are the best for me as they have some shape to them and they look better inside of your bra. As opposed to being a flat gauze / cotton pad.
Finally I bought little cold / hot packs for my girls. They are little circle donuts with ice / heat packs inside that you can freeze or

microwave. A good $15 investment I used them almost everyday and easy enough to put all of these items on your registry or use a $40 gift card and buy everything you need in the nipple care category. **$10-40**

10) Car Seat. They won't let you leave the hospital without a rear facing seat. There are high end ones, lower end ones, and this is something you want to buy new for your first baby then maybe recycle if you have another. The new rule is to keep them rear facing as long as possible, so buy a decent car seat that you are going to keep around for about 2 years. Make sure the pads remove easy so you can wash them, because you will have accidents and spills. Test it out at the store and I recommend getting one that has a base that stays in the car and a carrier that snaps out to tote your little one around in, though that is painfully heavy it can be convenient as a place for baby to sit if you are out and about. **$150-500**

At the end of the day this baby is going to eat, sleep and poop so be prepared for that. Also be prepared to try and keep the baby's body temperature pretty even. So appropriate levels and layers of clothing and light blankets are best.

Nice to have buy shop carefully:

It's a hard sell, but some of the below items unless gifted to you at your shower or you just had to have, you might want to wait a week and maybe keep them on your register or order them on line while you are home with baby. There are some big ticket items you might not need to spend all of the money on, especially if they are things that aren't going to work for you, your lifestyle or most importantly for your baby.

Nursing Pillow. I used regular pillows. I can see the advantage but by the 2nd baby I had nursing down and didn't need much assistance though the extra positioning help does take some of the strain off of your elbows, arms, etc. **$45**

Nursing Bras. Yes they make your life easier. They are ridiculously overpriced though and painfully ugly. Even the pretty ones. No underwires and soft no shape cups make them UGGGHH. I wear t-shirt bras and I need an underwire and a shaped cup. They are out there. I found some good cheap ones at Target. Clearance. You don't exactly need a matching bra and panty set for this task. I understand the comfort of the softcup and nice cotton but they look terrible. I found the nighttime nursing bras which are basically a cotton sports bra type thing completely useless. I wore my nursing bras out. I found that some days my boobs would fill up the cups and then some, spilling over the top. Other days, however, they would not, and that is NOT a good look having big divots in your bra visible through your shirt. So please note your cup size can fluctuate and change so it becomes even trickier and if you are only having one baby get a few nice ones but it's a tough investment to make for maybe a few months. **$20-60**

Breast Pump. I went all out the first time around and bought a really nice Philips Avent system with a hands free bra and extra storage bags. I used it less than a dozen times. It hurt me and I never got a good yield. Second time around I bought a manual hand pump. Which I used more than the Philips system and would pump every once in a while just to build a reserve. The manual pump while a little more labor intensive was infinitely simpler to use and quicker to implement. By the time you set up to pump with a dual hands free there is so much going on you might run out of time to actually pump. I've seen on TV the ones you can plug into the car charger and pump while driving – now that is brilliant for working moms. I would do that if I had had to go back to work right away. **$50 for a manual pump - $400**

Nursing Accessories In General. If you can hold off on buying them or get one bra and one tube of nipple cream and call it a day before the baby arrives. You don't know if you can breastfeed or not so before you drop about a grand on pumps, bras, pillows, etc. see if you can and if you want to. Some women just don't want to. Save your money, it's hard to return used pumps, bras, and pillows that a baby may or may not have barfed on. It's a drag but wait. Often the store you register with will issue you a one time sweep coupon of about 20% off to grab the last items on your registry. This is a perfect category to wait with. Or better yet if you get these items at your shower WAIT to open them so you can return them unused. It's hard before the baby comes not to open and look at and try and want to sterilize everything. You can wait. That week worth of patience could save you a lot of money on unused or not needed items that are in perfect shape so you can return them and get something you really need, like burp cloths and diapers.

Swaddling Cloths. A few of the simple cotton lightweight blankets that come in the multipacks will work just fine for the babies. The Velcro on the 'swaddling blankets / wraps" inevitably gets jacked up in the laundry no matter how careful you are. It catches on other clothes and renders the swaddling blankets useless at some point, non-functional and hopelessly misshapen after only a few washes. Plus you will find the big patches of Velcro will catch on and absolutely ruin any other semi delicate baby items. Learn how to swaddle in the hospital. **$15-20**

Baby Blankets. I had tons. Really I only needed 3 in different levels of warmth. My sister bought me an awesome microfiber lightweight blanket that served as a primary sleep cover after my baby girl was 6 months old. I have very thick ones that I never used. I have a whole drawer full that will eventually be doll blankets or end up in dog beds. Ehhh. Covers for the stroller rides. **$15-50**

Burp Cloths. The store bought ones I found to be while very cute and colorful aren't big or absorbent enough. Spit cloths to wipe up a little here and there, maybe. But when your child unleashes the full contents of their stomach all over themselves and you, it's not going to cut it. I used a few packs of cloth diapers and liked their texture and how light weight they are. The cheap cloth diaper packs, Carters or Gerber, are in the same section at the Target usually with the newborn white onesies. You can bleach them and they are decently absorbent. They aren't the cutest things going, but they work and you can throw them away when they get too messy. Sometimes it's hard to get rid of the cute stuff. **$10-15**

First Aid Kit. Yeah. It has all kinds of stuff. I don't know I didn't really use any of it. You need something to cut their little nails with, I used my own manicure scissors because I could handle them the best. Those kids are moving and don't want their little nails cut and sometimes the mini clippers in the kits just don't work as precisely as you need utilizing tired mommy hands on wiggly kids. You also need some type of plastic syringe or measured medicine doser for pain / fever relief and vitamins, though when you buy baby liquid medicines they usually have one included. Extras don't hurt. However I found the kits pretty worthless. **$20-40**

Baby Bathtub. Most of my friends swear by buying the foam petals for the sink and bathing baby in there. I received a bathtub as a gift and used it pretty religiously on both kids. Granted I didn't bathe my kids daily, but I found the tub useful in some ways and not in others. The pros are it's a contained unit with a cloth sling for the little ones and keeps them at a decent angle, etc. The cons are that it did not fit well on my countertop and I wanted to try and manage the kids at my height as much as possible versus bending over or kneeling on the ground. Too old for that. People my age are grandparents already. Once your child gets active it's hard to keep them in there, and I had tall skinny kids which made them a hard fit for all of the baby stuff. I put extra towels inside the tub for padding however that made the water get colder, faster. I found it easier in the long run to give the kids showers with me and I think the foam petals for the sink to use for the first few months then maybe a small blow up for the actual bathtub is the best bet.

Sleep Sound Generator And Nighttime Lotions. We have 2 sound generators. Used a few times. Ehh as most sleep aids for the babies I've found they work better on me then the kids since you are always on that cusp of really needing some good sleep. The lavender lotions and relaxing sounds can take you over the edge. I have a good friend who is a masseuse so I regularly massage my kids at night with nighttime lotion. I'm not sure it works. The lotion isn't that great either. The smell is strong and it's far from the best moisturizer I use on their skin. **$15-30**

Baby Monitor. We bought a very cheap one on clearance. One base and 2 receivers that can run on batteries or be plugged in. They are fine. There is lighted display that peaks with louder noises, like crying. I found myself using it very infrequently, more with my 2nd child then my first since I was running around after a toddler while the baby was napping. However you can hear your baby cry from a crazy distance away. For those of you who are hooked on video systems, that makes sense but really do you need to see the baby? Our house is 1800 sq. ft. Yes I can hear my babies cry from any and every room, and even when I'm outside. Jamie Sommers bionic hearing in play, doo doo doo doo doo. Hearing them cry then going to get them seems to be enough. **$30-200**

Things to make good investments in:

For all of the next items I suggest going to a store and look at the items. Push them around if they are strollers, try on carriers, touch the pack n play and stand next to a potential changing table to see if the height works for you. These are tactile purchases as much as you'd like to just shop on line for them, they are pivotal items in your daily routine and you need to touch and evaluate before you buy.

Pack N Play. Investing in a multi purpose *Pack N Play* will get you very far. In general their mattresses are pretty thin but there is an extra mattress type layer you can buy to add some padding. Get the tricked out one with the bassinet and changing station. You can't use those extras for very long, a month or two at most, but they help. You can't go wrong. If you don't want to buy a crib et. al for a while this totally works. We take it on trips to use in hotel rooms and I used to take one to work. The most versatile baby item you can buy. It's a play area, a place to sleep and with the infant features a changing table even. Plus with all of the color combinations available you can match any décor. We had 3 at one point. We kept 1 upstairs and 1 downstairs by the kitchen area. Hands down the most functional pieces of equipment you will ever buy and it can be used until they are big and or smart enough to figure out how to get out. Aside from changing their diapers and as a place to set them down to nap, sometimes you just need a safe containment spot while you clean or go to the bathroom or take a shower. I even decorated one of ours up with an extra little mobile and some extra padding. Worth it. Register for it. Once you get the hang of it you can put them up and take them down in only 1-2 minutes. The first one I bought was a discontinued pattern so I got a super deal on Amazon. It's the one in the picture. $45 shipped. After a bit of wear and tear I ended up taking that one and stationed it outside for my new baby when I'm out watching my son so she can get some fresh air and sunshine. Cleans up pretty easy. Love it. **$50-120**

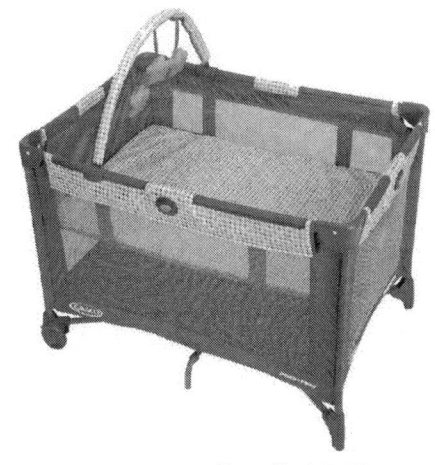

Graco Pack 'n Play

Changing Table. Find one that works for you. I missed the mark and bought a cheap one from Wal-Mart. The drawers started falling apart almost immediately. But I've used it through 2 kids mostly because it's the right height for me. I still use it to dress my 3 year old though he's painfully too tall and big for it. I am tall and I don't want to bend down to change diapers in the pack n play and I like my furniture too much to chance having an accident on it when taking a diaper on or off. I don't do poop anywhere other than a changing table. Heed that warning. Poop can get all over and out of control fast. My friend tells a story of her toddler having a poopie diaper being changed on her bed and her little one proceeded to put her hands in when mom took off her diaper and she crawled across the bed with the diaper in tow while mom was trying to get a handle on the situation. Not good. Even on the changing table things can go south very quickly. A quick grab of a poopie diaper, a shift, a sudden motion and boom you have poop everywhere and what became a routine diaper change is now a complete hose down and sterilization of an entire area and a load of laundry complete with scrubbing out poop and pre-soaking first. No thanks. As I'm winding down the baby stuff I'm less and less inclined to clean the poop out of anything. With a California water and energy crisis I do weigh the cost of the resources used to clean out a onesie or a towel versus buying a new one and buying a new one wins almost every single time.

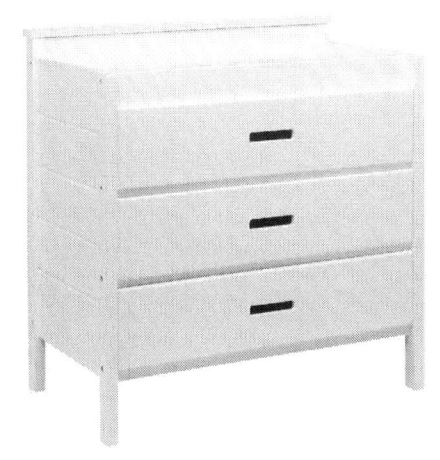

Walmart Baby Mod Modena 3 drawer changing table

High Chair. The item I had the most problems with but had to use 3 times a day every day. Make sure it comes up to a height that works for you. Make sure it's EASY TO CLEAN. Hello. I had a second hand high chair for my son. The chair pad was not removable so I cut it and put Velcro to seal it back up so I could take it off to clean it and throw it in the washer from time to time. Make sure it has a seatbelt and is mobile in some way. My old one had 4 wheels that you were supposed to lock down but I never did. My newest high chair is portable and folds up quickly, and from time to time I take my daughter outside to feed her. Stupidly the trays are different too. Some are easier to deal with than others.

Get a tray you can put in the dishwasher. Cleaning a tray is weird, mine don't really fit in my sink well and I feel wrong scrubbing it down with Windex when I really want to use soap and water. The tray liner is too easy for my little ones to remove and fling across the room they love doing so when it's full of food and my back is turned for a few seconds while I'm pouring a cup of coffee or feeding the dogs. I spend so much time cleaning this item and it never really gets clean. The tray and seat belt are caked in dried food that I have no hope of every scraping off properly. I clean my highchair 4-5 times a day. A scoop tray underneath would be awesome too. It just has too many nooks and crannies. The angles of the seat don't allow for a good cleaning and the drop off onto the floor is tremendous so I clean the floor a few times a day too. The one I have now the seat is at such an angle that the crumbs that accumulate fall right onto the floor which is annoying, whereas my old chair had a footrest that was big enough to catch the crumbs before they went on the ground. Get a high chair that lends its self to being hosed down too. I take it out in the backyard and hose it down every few weeks.

It really is the little details which you can't see until you already have it in your house and you are using it. They can be very expensive and while it makes sense to wait because you won't be using it for a while, if someone wants to spring for a high chair for your shower then let them.

If I could redesign high chairs this is what I would do;

- Adjustable height with a one foot range to fit everyone's needs. I like to sit and feed my daughter. I used to stand to feed my son. A foot lever in the back to go up or down.
- Wheels can be folded up into the legs like some bassinets.
- Non staining nylon padding comes up easily and can be washed in the washing machine or dishwasher.
- Both trays fit easily into a generic dishwasher.

- Reasonable Price. Come on. $500 is ridiculous. How about we all settle at $125. Even that seems high but we will load it up with all types of features.
- Easy Cleaning Seat. Designed in such a way that you can wipe the corners and wipe down to get all of the remnants without all of the food sticking in the seat corners then going onto the floor.
- Adjustable Foot rest. Tilts and adjusts like a dust pan to catch crumbs.

Travel System. I am very proud of two serious purchases I've made for my kids. The first was a travel system which consisted of a lockable wheel jog stroller, car seat and car seat base which stays in the car. Love it. Used it daily and used it again daily with my 2nd kid. We hike everyday on gravel trails and walk on the sidewalk. You want the front wheel to lock and unlock because when in the jogging position you cannot turn your stroller if the front wheel is locked. Great for jogging, even for actually walking around. I've written rave on line reviews of the system I purchased which I did by a seasonal coupon from Babies R Us plus I had it on my registry and got an extra discount when buying out remaining items so my total price was about $200. Very reasonable. I am also a huge fan of two piece infant car seat, with the separate base. So you have a carrier that you click into the base. Make sure the base is level, we made the mistake of not doing this quite right before we brought our first baby home. He was secure in the carrier section but the angle he was at in the car was off and made me nervous. I adjusted it the next day but it gave me stress. I bought neck stabilization pillows, never used them. They are like travel pillows for babies, ehhh I felt like it was too much behind them, on the back of their necks and made the angle in the seat weird. If the pillow just had bulk on either side of the head and not in the back it would be better and make more sense. Our carrier also had an infant insert, a pad that went around the perimeter that fastened via Velcro to the straps. We used that until the babies were big enough to not need it anymore. **$150 - 500**

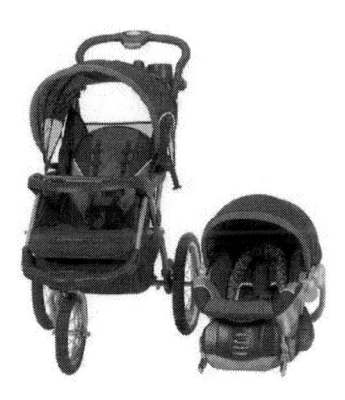

Baby Trend Expedition Travel System

Double Stroller. My 2nd awesome purchase. I researched this for months. I looked into purchase used ones and the higher end used ones were more expensive than the lower end new. I found one on special at Wal-Mart discounted because of it's color (it's red) and with a holiday special of free 2 day shipping my cost was $150. I love it. It has a lockable front wheel, snack tray (which many of the higher end units do not have) and I've heard that people steal the high end ones at theme parks all of the time. There are little parking lots you have to stow your stroller at when you are on rides and that people come and take them. Yikes. My Wal-mart version is slick looking, functional, turns well and I use it daily. The downsides are it's heavy, doesn't fold up small, and the under seat cargo bins don't hold much and they drag when they have stuff in them. I wasn't going to get one then I was so glad I did. My 3 year old wants to walk but is happy to ride from time to time. My 10 month old is comfy as can be.

All strollers have some of the same deficits and my neighbor swears by a cheap $25 dollar umbrella fold up from Target vs. the higher end ones. No stroller really folds down well. It's hard to get in the trunk of a car. We have an SUV and we lose the whole back with the double stroller. The typical high end units and high end joggers have fixed wheels and no snack tray. Not for me. Both my single and double have the lockable front wheel so you can walk or run. If you run with the wheels unlocked it's not good.

The stroller vibrates to a ridiculous degree and you lose control. When the wheel is locked you lose the ability to steer and have to go straight but you can run without issue. I don't really run but this design works best for me and I need snack trays. My 3 year old will eat his morning or afternoon snack while my little one sleeps while I push them both up and down hills in my neighborhood to get exercise.

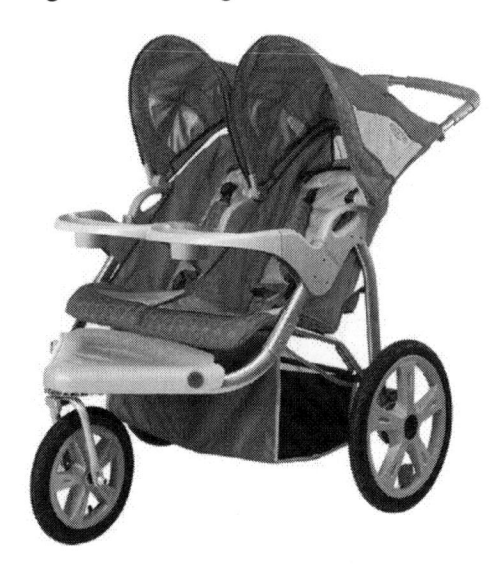

InStep Safari Double Jogging Stroller

Now my neighborhood has the have and the have nots. The $1000 expensive high end strollers are prevalent. I also see them for sale all over the local web sites and selling channels. For hundreds and hundreds of dollars. A little word of advice. Especially if you live in a family neighborhood. Your light use, clean non smoking house $1000 stroller and high end furniture isn't worth anything on the resale market. Good luck. Better off donating it all and taking the deduction. For real. Or sell it for $150 not $500. The lower you price your precious baby items, that you paid way too much for and didn't get nearly the amount of use to justify the cost of them for, the more likely you are to actually sell them. Used items aren't worth a fixed percentage of the new or replacement cost, they are worth what someone is willing to pay and most parents in affluent neighborhoods aren't going to buy a used anything for their precious babies and the not so affluent neighborhoods aren't going to buy your $1500 convertible crib you are 'sacrificing' to sell for only $800. You don't always have to buy the best. The kids are going to thrash all of your nice things. My $150 Wal-Mart special discontinued color double stroller is now one year old and I use it every single day. It's holding up fine. It's dirty and stained and the tread on the tires is worn down but it's totally functional and I've gotten every penny out of it and the kids have loved it and I'm going to donate it and take the tax deduction. So suck on that with your BOB deluxe high end double. **$150-1000**

Baby Carrier. I received 2 at my shower and used them so often that by the time I went put them in the charity pile I almost threw them away. They were stained with sweat and dirt. Very well used. Take some time to shop for this. There are so many price ranges and styles. Some like the Moby wraps are giant cloth strips that you weave around your body. I used the ones that were like mini backpacks for the baby. If you can go to a store where you can try them on, or if you get one or more from your shower TRY IT ON and put a dog or something in there. Seriously. You want to find one that supports your lower back and doesn't destroy your neck and shoulders. The one I had that I loved and used the most was from Target. About $50. I thought I used it quite a bit with my first baby. I used to take him for walks in it every day before he was old enough and big enough to sit by himself in the stroller without the infant car seat. I used it at the grocery store because I was afraid to put the infant car seat in the grocery cart after reading an article about how unsafe it was. That was nothing compared to how often I used it after my daughter was born. Chasing after a toddler requires 2 hands so my baby ended up in that carrier constantly. When we were walking, at the store, and even around the house. I found with both kids that the carrier can be considered a workout essential as well. For walking and hiking, I used it all of the time to get exercise for myself. Adding the extra 10 -25 pounds (my max with the carrier, it taxed my back too much to have a heavier, tall kid in it and I never felt comfortable flipping it around to be like a backpack) really gets the blood pumping and the sweat flowing. **$40-200**

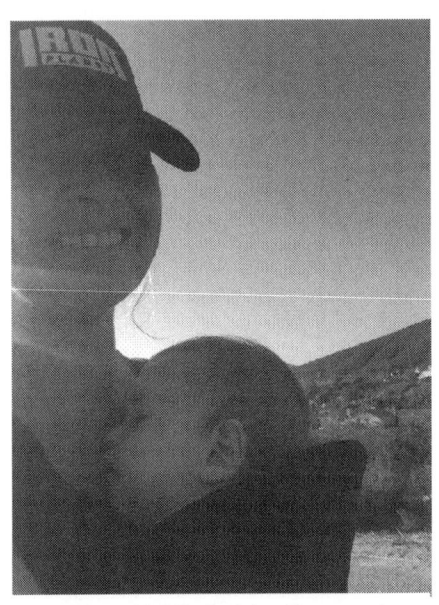

Walking with Elizabeth in a front carrier

Baby Lotion and Oils. I suggest spending decent money here. The cheap ones are usually pink, or purple for the nighttime calming ones. Between the scent and the coloring they are overwhelming and make me gag so find yourself a decently priced lotion that you will love and have no problem putting on baby over and over again. Some recommend coconut oil, if you like it, buy it. I found a moderately priced brand over at Babies R Us that had 2 types I really liked; one was infused with a natural orange scent and the other had an olive oil base. Both were white, lightly scented, and effective. There are some very pricey lotions on the market, find what you can live with but this is your kids skin so spend a few extra bucks. Oils are a tougher sell. I used them occasionally when their skin got super dry, however better as a make up remover than a moisturizer. Like lip balms I found the more oil I used, the drier their skin got. Stick with a simple lotion you can put on everyday after baths or while getting them dressed. **$8-20**

And into the first year:

Exercauser. There are a few different types. Ones that are like a giant saucer and ones that are more like a bungee chair. I got one from my baby shower and I definitely got good use out of it on both kids. It's a useful unit for keeping the kids in one place. Unlike a walker they aren't going anywhere and there are usually some toys on it and a snack tray. The downside is that the seats are HUGE and I always had to put extra padding in the form of a folded up towel behind the kids to support them. By the time the kids would grow big enough to fill up the seat they will have outgrown the height. I have tall slender kids and most toys and clothing accommodate shorter stockier infants and toddlers. My daughter outgrew the height on the walker and exercauser by the time she was 9 months old. In sum if you get one free, take it, register for it, but buy it later if you think it will be useful. **$60**

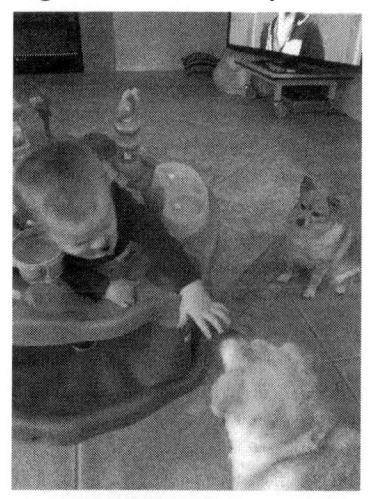

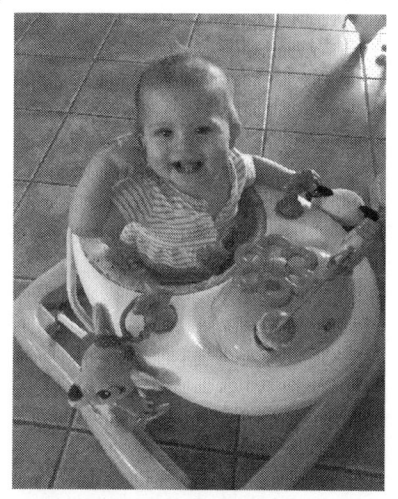

Jacob in his exercauser   Elizabeth in her pink walker

Walker. I have been blessed with tall kids. Kids who before they can really walk can topple over in the standard walkers. I set them right away at the max height and they are still too small. I like that it get's them moving and their little legs mobile however did you know that they are banned in Canada. I'm not familiar with the language of the law but the philosophy is that they are dangerous. Yes they certainly can be. This is a DOWNSTAIRS unit only, not for use anywhere near stairs, ledges, lips, anything other than smooth even floor with no step downs. I also understand the thought is that they delay the development of walking. Interesting. I recently saw a blurb about buying a large blow up pool and plopping it in your living area for the baby to hang out in. Looks kind of cool too. I used walkers. They were fine. Kids liked them. They would even take the dogs for rides too. Super dangerous stuff. **$25-60**

General Purchasing Advice:

Clothing. My first baby I was grossed out by the thought of having my son's stomach hanging out so I had him in onesies and one piece pajamas for the first year and a half. Oh and socks. Always socks. It was 70 degrees outside and he would have fleece pants, a long sleeved onesie and socks. What an idiot I was. He also looked super dorky. I did my best but I look back and my choices weren't the greatest. I have a neighbor who swears by PJ's and her kids are always in either footie Phi's or 2 piece sets. As a stay at home mom that is super practical. Two pieces are much much easier to change diapers with, top and bottom. Don't buy too many clothes in advance. Your friends will do it for you. Predicting that first size is also super tricky. Don't buy P's (preemies size) and if the baby is going to be decent sized you might want to start at the 3 month

Also there is a benefactor train that you might end up on. When my daughter was on her way, a friend of mine sent a giant box of clothes. I was the first one since she had her little girl to have another girl in our group of friends. Score. It had clothes for the first year and took the pressure of me to acquire clothing except for special outfits or things I just couldn't live without. I've gifted hundreds of outfits to friends over the years, as they grow so fast their light use clothes and especially my kids shoes for the first year or two were in such perfect shape I was able to pass them along to a friend who has a son a year younger than mine.

My kids go through 2-3 outfits a day without accidents. With accidents and getting dirty playing its more like 4-5. Be prepared. Target has Carters cotton pants in a double pack for less than $10 and tons of t-shirts under $5. We stock up at Target and Old Navy when there are sales. If you hit a great sale at Old Navy plus clearance you can really score on everything from shirts to Phi's to nice pants and particularly flip flops. I buy clothes at Target once a month for each kid. I hunt for clearance and out of season items. I buy clothes at Old Navy once a quarter trying to match up with their super sales. They stay in most of their clothes for such a short period of time so I don't care if I buy things that are built to last, I make sure they have plenty of clothes to play in and look decent and are fun. Remember to have fun. Solids are great for adults. Fun clothes are best for kids. Play clothes. Costumes even. Target has such amazing and inexpensive licensed items that my kids love. Old Navy is great for the solids and basics and jeans and jackets, especially jackets. For the little kids Old Navy is awesome for multi packs of onesies, t-shirts and socks.

As of late I've found that Wal-Mart is coming on strong too. Their prices are really low, clothing is ok holds up decently, usually has some cool licensed character shirts (which as much as you want your stylish kids to look fly at some point they want a Batman or a Paw Patrol shirt) and lasts about as long as you need it to. I just read that Wal-Mart is taking a new strategy to try and compete with Amazon and I've found that they type of feedback they are looking for after purchase is in line with that. They are offering a ton more via their website and app from various 3rd party vendors. I made my last 2 big buys for my little girl via the iphone app. Cute stuff. For around $65 I purchased a set of 'it's getting colder in San Diego' wardrobe consisting of 2 hoodies, 3 long sleeved shirts, 4 leggings and a pair of super stylist Jordache jeans with glitter in the fabric. She loves them. Wants to wear them everyday.

I find that clothing was always about 3 distinct waves. One, I would try to buy clothes a season or size a head on sale when I could. That way I was stocking and prepared. There are many times where your child grows overnight. You wake up and they don't fit into their pants anymore. I have had this happen to me so many times, where we are in shorts for a few weeks because it's hot then when I need a pair of pants they are too short and the waist is too small. Time to move into the next size and I always find comfort in having a few basics in the next size cued up and to have purchased them on sale or clearance makes me feel good too. I don't like spending a lot on clothes, mostly because they get destroyed or grown out of so quickly. The second wave of purchase for me would be to fill in the gaps. I do laundry pretty regularly and it becomes quickly apparent what you are short on. Long sleeved shirts, long pants, shorts, short sleeved shirts, socks. Its not fun to feel like you don't have a good reserve. The balance is to not have too many of one category because inevitably as soon as you get more than enough you wont need them anymore. The final wave is specialty clothes for holidays or going to an event. I find myself picking up a pair of shoes that maybe only will get worn once with a Christmas dress or fancy outfit. Some occasions warrant this, sometimes it feels like a waste. A nice pair of holiday shoes to match the fabulous outfit you bought will run you $15-25. For that you can buy 5-8 everyday basic items from the Wal-Mart.

I'm doing a much better job dressing my second. It's your taste getting imprinted on a little one. I like to be light and whimsical and practical. They are kids, not accountants or gothic graphic artists. I love bright and frilly and fun for my little girl, and I love tough and practical with lots of character themes for my little boy. He is either in a Spiderman shirt, some type of sports team or theme, something with a picture of a construction vehicle, or his favorite super hero. Cotton pants and shorts are a must for him, as he's growing I find shorts the much more practical choice, a lesson learned in the 3T size where I had loads of pants that became obsolete overnight. Living in San Diego, shorts and a t-shirt are the accepted look all of the time, you can never go wrong with the little surfer boy look of some board shorts and a shirt. My little girl gets color, color and more color. Pink, red, purple, greens, tons of mix and match color. I use gray, black and white as neutral pieces for leggings and some tops but I always have some color or point of interest on her clothes. They are only this little once, and having a 9 year old I can tell you there comes a time where they don't want your choices or input anymore so dress them while you can. I bought a few of those really cute animal themed bunting outfits when they were babies, Old Navy has a white fleece one piece with feet and a hood that looks like a bear. So cute. My daughter wore that on her first Halloween. So many cute hoodies and Phi's so just go for it and have fun!!!

New Versus Used. If I knew now, I would put my money into different areas. I would solicit friends a bit more too. I ended up gifting so many awesome items that were in great shape. Just recently as I'm ending the infant stages of my kids and moving into little kids and toddlers exclusively I gave away a lightly used dual electric breast pump, a high end diaper bag, cute holiday outfits and warm up suits, storage bottles, and this was all to someone I met once who happened to need these items at the time I was trying to figure out the best way to get rid of them. A lot of what you need or want for that first year to year and a half doesn't get you into the toddler years. They outgrow it or it becomes impractical.

There are also baby item swap meets and discount bazaar's, the yoga studio I used to go to was attached to a high end baby boutique that now also houses a birthing center. They have a street fair type of swap every few months with strollers, clothes, all kinds of things. We live in San Diego and there are several very affluent communities within 20 miles of us. That is where you want to tap into for used items. If you want to buy a super high end stroller look into nextdoor.com or one of the other online apps that have close radius private sales similar to garage sales.

Items I Regret Not Having. Only a few. I wish I had invested in one of those cradle rocker glider things. They are about $150 and I wish I had bought that instead of the swing / bounce chair and some other items. I felt compelled to use a basinet we had from my husband's first child, I cleaned it up and bought a new mattress and it was pretty so I wanted to use it but I wish instead of being practical about that one piece I had bought the cradle rocker instead. I wish I had even picked up a used one and given it the same TLC as our hand me down basinet. My neighbor has the higher end one that adjusts into kind of a seating position and it oscillates and it's amazing.

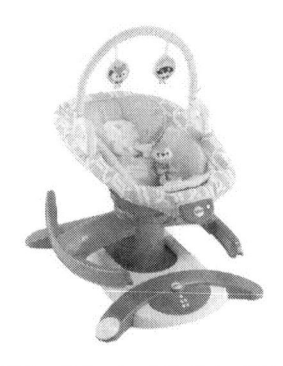

Fisher Price 4-n-1 Rock 'n Glide Soother

I also wish I had bought one of those slings where you could put your baby on your boob, swaddle them in and go hands free. Hands free is so important with baby #2 I can't even tell you. You need both hands to keep your toddler from flying off the counter, swimming in the toilet or lighting the house on fire. How awesome is that. I wish I had bought one. I had a friend who bought one of those complicated carriers like is like 10 feet of cloth that you have to figure out how to wrap around you.

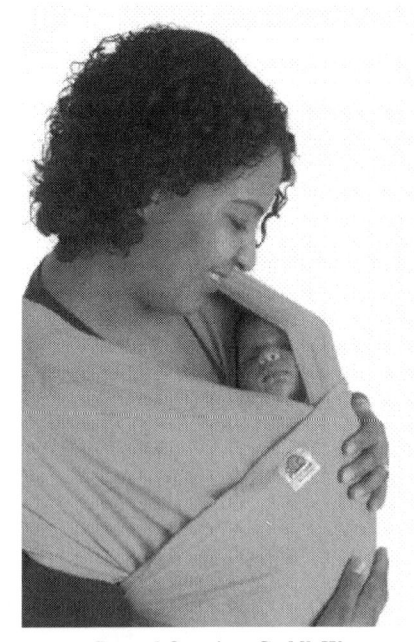

Peapod Creations CuddlyWrap

Tips For Your Registry And Your Shower (If You Have One.)
A few bits of insight about your shower. Whatever you need to take back after the shower because you have duplicates (yes it happens even with a list and a registry) use to buy your essentials. Target takes back items with no issues. Babies R Us is a bit trickier, as is Buy Buy Baby. You will have things to take back that you can convert into a gift card.

Request gift cards instead of items. Registering for things like baby bottles might get you something that 4-6 months down the line your kid might not like or want to use.

Finally it's all about how easy something is to clean. You spend a lot of time cleaning and cleaning and cleaning again as a new parent. The easier something is to clean the better. The more it will preserve your sanity.

I highly recommend if you register at Target or something similar that you add a stain removal system to your list. Either a Spot Bot or a steam mop. You will need it.

Finally keep it all as simple as possible. Easy for you to manage, easy for you to maintain, easy for you to use. The baby will be happy with whatever you provide, trust me. Can you throw it in the wash? Perfect. How about throw it in the dishwasher? Even better. It's hard to be ungrateful for a gift for a new baby but after our daughter was born we received a very expensive onesie. Sweater material, purple and white striped but it had TWO DOZEN miniature buttons to get it on and off. NFW!!! I put it on once and it came off at the next changing and went into the donation pile. I prided myself on sending every gift giver a picture of our kid in the item they gave us, but that one only lasted a minute. I was too tired, my fingers too clumsy to even try and manage dealing with something like that. That's why people love sleep sacks, easy on easy off. They weren't my taste but they are sure convenient. You'll find that mostly when people want to gift you it goes ones of two ways: they want you to ooh and aah over their exquisite taste, or they buy you something that they really think you need.

The simpler, the better. You will be tired. You will be exhausted. You will not want to mess around with putting something together or using something so complicated or hard to clean that it takes you over the edge of being a tired but happy mom into the kraken who wants to rage down like Godzilla on anything, usually your husband or partner btw, that gets in your way. I have thrown and kicked inanimate objects out of frustration. I have taken toys, clothes all kinds of things and chucked them in the garbage. Adulting is hard, parenting is atomic bomb level difficult. Your kids will survive without the latest and the greatest. Keep them as clean as you can, keep them safe, keep them warm and you are well on your way to another happy day in paradise.

Printed in Poland
by Amazon Fulfillment
Poland Sp. z o.o., Wrocław